The Megaloblastic Anaemias

I. CHANARIN MD, FRCPath

MRC Clinical Research Centre
and Northwick Park Hospital,
Harrow, Middlesex

THIRD EDITION

BLACKWELL SCIENTIFIC PUBLICATIONS

OXFORD LONDON

EDINBURGH BOSTON MELBOURNE

© 1969, 1979, 1990 by
Blackwell Scientific Publications
Editorial Offices:
Osney Mead, Oxford OX2 0EL
25 John Street, London WC1N 2BL
23 Ainslie Place, Edinburgh EH3 6AJ
3 Cambridge Center, Suite 208
  Cambridge, Massachusetts 02142,
  USA
107 Barry Street, Carlton
  Victoria 3053, Australia

First published 1969
Second edition 1979
Third edition 1990

Set by Best-Set Typesetter Ltd,
Hong Kong
Printed and bound in Great Britain
at The University Press, Cambridge

DISTRIBUTORS

Marston Book Services Ltd
PO Box 87
Oxford OX2 0DT
(*Orders*: Tel. 0865 791155
       Fax: 0865 791927
       Telex: 837515)

USA
  Year Book Medical Publishers
  200 North LaSalle Street
  Chicago, Illinois 60601
  (*Orders*: Tel: (312) 726-9733)

Canada
  The C.V. Mosby Company
  5240 Finch Avenue East
  Scarborough, Ontario
  (*Orders*: Tel: (416) 298-1588)

Australia
  Blackwell Scientific Publications
  (Australia) Pty Ltd
  107 Barry Street
  Carlton, Victoria 3053
  (*Orders*: Tel: (03) 347-0300)

British Library
Cataloguing in Publication Data

Chanarin, I. (Isreal)
  The megaloblastic anaemias. —
  3rd ed
  I. Man. Blood.
  Megaloblastic anaemia
  I. Title
  616.1'52

ISBN 0-632-02549-2

Contents

Preface to the third edition

The earlier editions of *The Megaloblastic Anaemias*, appearing in 1969 and 1979, were relatively large volumes which reviewed the field in some depth. The third edition is much smaller. It contains some 437 references as compared to 4258 in the second edition, and these largely refer to work published since 1980. The text, however, is complete in itself and while describing the common disorders contains new sections reflecting increased understanding of inherited disorders of cobalamin metabolism and of less common disorders which have now become much better defined. As in earlier editions the physiology of cobalamin and folates is described and the criteria which should be used in assessing and managing deficiency states are discussed. This volume should be regarded as complementary to the detailed accounts of the field in the earlier editions.

Preface to the first edition

My principal object in writing a preface is to acknowledge my indebtedness to many friends who have helped me in the preparation of this book and permitted me to reproduce material from their own work.

I am deeply grateful to Dr Leo Duchen for the magnificent photographs of the spinal cord changes in vitamine B_{12} neuropathy; Dr C.A. Finch for permission to reproduce his now classical illustrations of the changes in iron metabolism in pernicious anaemia; Dr P. Hoedemaeker for the elegant autoradiographs illustrating the localization of intrinsic factor to the gastric parietal cell; Dr J.W. Laws for the photographs of the X-ray appearance of the normal and pernicious anaemia stomach; Dr Humphrey Lloyd for the photographs of the changes in the epithelium of the cervix uteri in megaloblastic anaemia; Dr Jerry Trier for the excellent illustration of the changes in the jejunal mucosa in untreated pernicious anaemia; Dr E.H. Reynolds for allowing me to publish his observations on folate levels in the CSF in epilepsy and, not least, Dr Leon Szur for his very helpful advice on the section on the isotopes of vitamin B_{12}.

I am particularly indebted to Miss Janet Perry, who not only read the proofs, but also checked the larger number of references in the text and, with Miss W. Gallagher, showed an uncanny skill in tracing obscure references. Miss Suzanne Okholm, Mrs Ann Jones, Mrs Inge Barnett and others patiently typed and retyped the manuscript and finally I am grateful to the forbearance of my colleagues who shouldered a larger proportion of routine chores than usual during the preparation of this book.

Every attempt has been made to make correct attribution to the many recorded observations in this complex field. It is likely, however, that important observations may have been overlooked particularly in the case of papers in languages other than English. I must express my regrets in advance for such omissions and indicate that they are entirely inadvertent.

Chapter 1   Introduction

Megaloblastic anaemia is a common disorder encountered in daily haematological practice. The possibility of such a diagnosis needs to be considered with every blood count showing an increase in red cell size. Throughout the world folate deficiency is common in inadequately nourished populations and may affect half the pregnant women in such countries [1]. Pernicious anaemia, the common form of cobalamin deficiency, affects more than 1% of older persons. Nevertheless, the investigation of these problems is increasingly a lost art.

The pressures accompanying the management of patients with leukaemia has led to decreasing interest in other blood disorders. The simple elucidation of the cause of megaloblastic anaemia is poorly done, criteria on which diagnosis is made are often inadequate and conclusions reached are often incorrect.

An evaluation of the response of physicians to a report of a low serum cobalamin following a request which they had initiated was adequate in only one-third of patients, and in more than 40% of 250 patients the report was ignored [2].

Definitions   The megaloblast is an abnormal red cell precursor in the marrow which differs from the normoblast, the normal red cell precursor, in several respects. It is larger than its normal counterpart, the nuclear pattern in fixed and stained preparations tends to be finely stippled as contrasted with coarser clefts in the normoblast nucleus and it tends to retain cytoplasmic basophilia as the cell matures. This form of haemopoiesis is termed megaloblastic.

In addition to changes in erythroblasts there are abnormal white blood cells. In the marrow, granulocyte precursors tend to be larger than their normal counterparts but the most striking change is the presence of large metamyelocytes with a horseshoe-shaped nucleus — termed a giant metamyelocyte.

Morphological changes in megakaryocytes are more dif-

1

ficult to recognize, but abnormal nuclear patterns as in megaloblasts may be seen in severe megaloblastic anaemia.

In the peripheral blood the common feature is an increase
in red cell size, termed macrocytosis, seen on inspection of a
stained peripheral blood film, and an increased mean corpuscular volume (MCV) when a blood count is carried out. In
addition the well-developed case shows a small number of
neutrophil polymorphs with an increased number of nuclear
lobes.

Megaloblastic changes are also detectable in other tissues
such as skin, buccal, vaginal and uterine cervical cells and in
macrophages such as those in the lungs. These cells are larger
than normal with a finely stippled nuclear chromatin.

Diagnosis of megalobastosis is based entirely on the
recognition of these changes in well-spread and well-fixed
peripheral blood and marrow preparations. There is no other
way by which such a diagnosis can be established. Haematinics given prematurely, either as therapy or as part of diagnostic tests, may restore normoblastic haemopoiesis, and if
adequate material for diagnosis has not been collected, may
make it very difficult or impossible to reach a proper diagnosis.

The clinical importance of megaloblastic anaemia is that
it is commonly due to a deficiency of either folate or cobalamin, and therapy with the appropriate vitamin produces
very gratifying clinical benefits. Cobalamin deficiency too can
cause a severe neuropathy and if treated in the earlier stages
is almost completely reversible. Although a clinical suspicion
of megaloblastic anaemia may initiate appropriate investigations, diagnosis must be made in the laboratory from examination of the blood and marrow.

Megaloblastosis can also be due to a variety of drugs or to
rare inborn errors of metabolism.

These aspects, the pathophysiology of megaloblastic states
and the peculiar features of cobalamin and folate that make deficiency so common are considered in the following chapters.

Chapter 2 Clinical presentation in megaloblastic anaemia

Signs and symptoms in cobalamin deficiency

There are many causes of cobalamin (Cbl) deficiency but the consequences are similar in the majority of patients although nuances vary with different aetiological factors.

On occasion patients are detected for the first time by the finding of macrocytosis on a blood count. Some such patients may have few complaints. More commonly, however, patients present because of weariness and lethargy (90%), shortness of breath (50%), tingling in hands and/or feet (30%) and a sore mouth or tongue (20%). The onset of symptoms is gradual and the average duration of symptoms exceeds 1 year before the patient seeks medical attention. Symptoms due to anaemia are tiredness, dyspnoea on exertion, palpitations and, with severe anaemia, signs of congestive cardiac failure and angina on effort.

Loss of appetite and even anorexia may explain weight loss. A sore mouth and tongue is a common feature, being present intermittently, and may be aggravated by certain foods. Dentures may be too painful to wear. Loss of taste or the presence of unusual tastes may occur. Some complain of dyspeptic symptoms. Diarrhoea is relatively uncommon.

Changes in skin and hair pigmentation, particularly in non-Caucasian patients, occur. Brown pigmentation about finger and toe nails disappearing with therapy has been noted in Indian patients. Loss of hair pigmentation may be restored by Cbl therapy (Fig. 2.1). Premature greying of hair and even alopecia is described.

Impotence is not uncommon and infertility in both sexes is the rule.

Cobalamin neuropathy

The commonest and usually the first symptom of nervous system involvement in Cbl deficiency is paraesthesiae, such as a tingling sensation in fingers and/or toes or numbness. The distribution of these symptoms is always symmetrical. There may be spastic movements, stiffness and weakness.

3

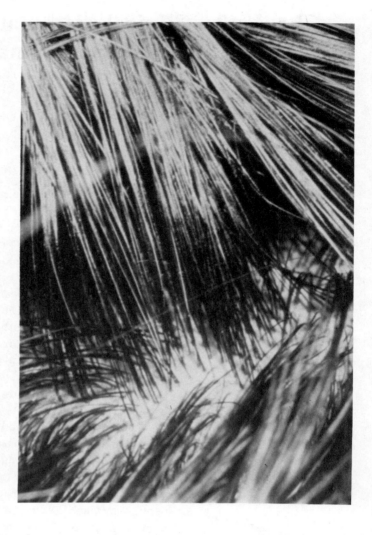

Fig. 2.1 Scalp hair of a 19-year Indian vegetarian with severe megaloblastic anaemia 3 months after treatment with oral Cbl. At presentation his hair colour was a dingy grey. After Cbl treatment normal black pigmentation was restored. The photograph shows the post-treatment black hair and pre-treatment grey hair.

Lhermitte's sign may be positive. Genito-urinary problems may be the result of neuropathy. Difficulties with micturition include hesitancy, poor urinary stream and even urinary retention. Constipation and postural hypotension may be due to the involvement of the autonomic nervous system.

Irritability, memory disturbance, mild depression and fluctuations of mood are present in a quarter to over half the patients with untreated pernicious anaemia. Rarely apathy, stupor, hallucinations, both auditory and visual, and even agitation and maniacal behaviour may occur.

Impairment and even loss of vision is an unusual manifestation. Such patients complain of a gradually failing vision and difficulty in reading small print.

Signs   Pallor combined with a lemon-yellow tint due to mild icterus is present in more anaemic Caucasian patients. A smooth shiny tongue even in the absence of a sore mouth is usual in pernicious anaemia. There may be painful cracks at the angles of the mouth. Others have a red beefy tongue.

Skin pigmentation and loss of hair pigment has been mentioned. Alopecia can occur. Vitiligo is a not uncommon accompaniment of pernicious anaemia. Pyrexia in more anaemic cases is common, without any detectable source of infection.

In severe anaemia there is tachycardia and a low blood pressure. A soft systolic murmur may be present on auscultation. Severe cases may be in cardiac failure with distended neck veins, ankle oedema and cardiac enlargement. The liver may be palpable but splenomegaly is rare.

Patients presenting with symptoms of neuropathy may not have any demonstrable abnormality in the early stages. More usually there is impairment of touch, temperature appreciation, and pain in the distal limbs at first and extending up the arms and legs. There is often loss of vibration sense, appreciation of passive movement and a positive Romberg's sign. Involvement of the lateral columns of the spinal cord produces exaggerated knee jerks and an extensor plantar. But some have a flaccid paralysis due to concomitant peripheral nerve and posterior column involvement. Muscle wasting may be present. Those with urinary difficulty may have an atonic bladder.

Of 14 patients with psychiatric manifestations, all had pronounced mental slowness, confusion and a memory defect, half were depressed, one-third had delusions, auditory or visual, one had parasitophobia and one extreme agitation and violent behaviour. Most of these patients had spinal cord involvement with severe anaemia.

Visual impairment may be due to haemorrhage in the macular region usually in thrombocytopenic patients. Retrobulbar neuritis (optic atrophy) is uncommon (about 0.3% of all pernicious anaemia patients) and males preponderate; 26 out of 29 patients with optic atrophy were men [3]. The optic discs may show pallor involving the whole disc or just the temporal side. There is contraction of the visual field and all cases have bilateral centrocaecal scotomata. There is impaired colour vision.

A neuropsychiatric study in 50 patients with megaloblastic anaemia due to Cbl deficiency showed that one-third were normal and the most common abnormality in 40% was peripheral neuropathy indicated by paraesthesia, absent reflexes and impaired vibration sense mainly in the legs. A further 25% showed abnormal nerve conduction on electrophysiological testing, although there was no clinical abnormality. Subacute combined degeneration of the cord was present in 16% of patients accompanied by evidence of peripheral neuropathy. An affective disorder as assessed by interview and self-rating scales was present in 20% of patients. One out of 50 had optic atrophy [4].

Signs and symptoms in folate deficiency

The signs and symptoms due to anaemia are the same in both Cbl and folate deficiency. The impairment of cell renewal, present when there is megaloblastic haemopoiesis, not only gives rise to anaemia but to changes in the epithelial surfaces so that a smooth and sometimes sore tongue and mouth may be present in folate deficiency as well as in Cbl deficiency.

The underlying cause of the folate deficiency may make its contribution to the clinical presentation although in other cases it may be silent. A patient with coeliac disease may have no symptoms and signs pertaining to intestinal malabsorption while others have a history of bulky stools and have short stature, etc. Both may have equally severe anaemia and megaloblastosis.

Depression is a not uncommon accompaniment of folate deficiency. An affective disorder, generally, depression was present in 19 of 34 patients with megaloblastic anaemia due to folate deficiency [4]; weakness or ataxia was present in two, paraesthesia in two and absent ankle jerks in three. Two patients among the 34 had impaired vibration sense and one impaired joint position sense. Although none in this small series of patients with folate deficiency had subacute combined degeneration of the cord Pincus and others [5] have described such cases. Reduced or absent sensory nerve potentials in patients receiving anticonvulsant drugs who had peripheral neuropathy and low serum and cerebrospinal fluid folate levels have been reported. These were reversed after treatment with folic acid or 5-formyltetrahydrofolate, the latter being the more effective [6]. Nevertheless, evidence of a neuropathy in a patient with macrocytosis points to Cbl deficiency as the likely reason, and Cbl deficiency must be excluded before serious consideration can be given to folate deficiency as a cause.

Haematology in megaloblastic anaemia

The effect of Cbl or folate deficiency is most marked in replicating cells. Thus the greatest effect is usually on the blood and thereafter on epithelial tissues undergoing cell renewal such as skin, gut mucosa and genito-urinary surfaces. Ultimately the effect is on all three major haemopoietic cell lines: red cells, white cells and platelets. In early disease only changes in red cells are detectable. The earliest and most consistent effect of Cbl or folate deficiency is in increasing cell size. In red cells this is a macrocytosis and the mean corpuscular volume (MCV) is raised above the normal range (Figs 2.2 and 2.3).

The normal range for MCV determined on automated cell counters varies in different institutions. Generally 80 femtolitres (fl) is accepted as the lower limit of the normal range. The upper limit ranges from 90 to over 100 fl. This variation reflects the absence of any absolute standard, problems posed by machine setting (does one make an adjustment for trapped

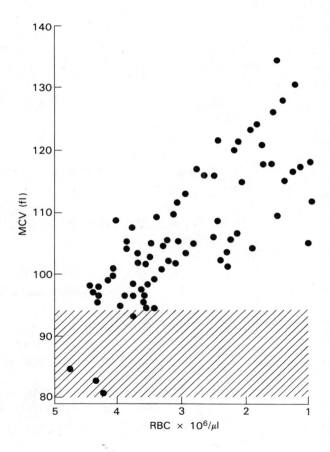

Fig. 2.2 The mean corpuscular volume and red cell count in untreated pernicious anaemia. The hatched area indicates the normal range.

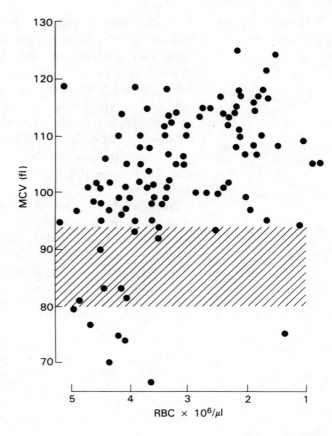

Fig. 2.3 The MCV and red cell
count in Hindu vegetarian
patients with megaloblastic
anaemia. There is a high
frequency of accompanying iron
deficiency due to poor availability
of iron from a vegetarian diet and
thalassaemia trait. These
conditions produce small red
blood cells. When such patients
develop a megaloblastic anaemia
the MCV may be either normal or
even below the normal range.
The hatched area indicates the
normal range.

plasma since the MCV is the haematocrit divided by the red
cell count?), and possibly populations used in establishing a
normal range. The range is much tighter when healthy adults
are used (80–90 fl) but patients include a significant number
with MCVs between 90 and 100 fl for which no ready explanation is available.

Macrocytosis   Macrocytosis (or a raised MCV), other than that due to Cbl or
folate deficiency, is associated with the following.
    Alcoholism.
    Hypothyroid states.
    Young red cell population including:
        chronic haemolysis, congenital and acquired,
        response to blood loss.
    Congenital dyshaemopoietic anaemias.
    Myelodysplastic syndromes including:
        primary sideroblastic anaemia;

5Q syndrome;
smouldering myelo-monocytic leukaemia.
Neoplasia.
Drugs including:
    hydroxyurea, methotrexate, 5-fluorouracil;
    cytosine arabinoside;
    6-mercaptopurine and thioguanine;
    anticonvulsants;
    melphalan.
Acquired marrow failure (aplastic and hypoplastic anaemia).
Liver failure.
Down's syndrome.
Chronic airways disease.
Familial (?).
Copper deficiency.
Diabetic ketoacidosis.
Physiological including:
    newborn;
    pregnancy.
Orotic aciduria.
Lesch–Nyhan syndrome.
Hairy cell leukaemia.
Cold agglutinins.
Unexplained in mature women (?hormonal).
Artefactual in blood samples left at room temperature for
    several hours.
Unexplained.

It is clear therefore that megaloblastic anaemia will account for only a small proportion of patients with abnormally large red cells, although the larger the red cells the more probable it is that the diagnosis is likely to be megaloblastosis.

Megaloblastosis with a normal or low MCV

Abnormally small red cells (microcytosis) occurs in the following.
    Iron deficiency.
    Thalassaemia syndromes.
    Anaemia of chronic disorders.
    Hyperthyroidism.
When such patients develop additional Cbl or folate deficiency with megaloblastosis, the size of the red cells increases generally into the normal range (Fig. 2.4). It is thus difficult to suspect megaloblastosis in the first instance. When anaemia is relatively severe, bizarre red cell fragments with hypersegmented neutrophils appear in peripheral blood films. In al-

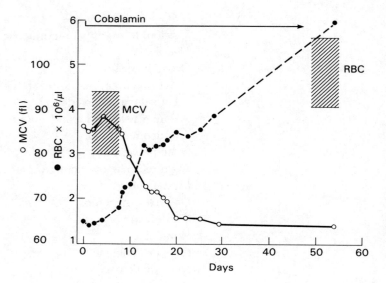

Fig. 2.4 The haematological changes in a patient with both pernicious anaemia and β-thalassaemia trait. On presentation the MCV was normal. However, on treatment with Cbl the MCV rose initially and thereafter fell to 64 fl being the value expected in thalassaemia trait. Likewise the red cell count rose from 1.5 × 10^6/μl to 6.0 × 10^6/μl. The hatched areas indicate the normal range.

most all cases the marrow will be megaloblastic. In others the suspicion of a megaloblastic component emerges as the anaemia is investigated. Thus administration of iron to a patient with both iron and Cbl or folate deficiency will result in the emergence of a macrocytic red cell population and an increase in the MCV (Fig. 2.5). The possibility of thalassaemia may be suggested by the patients' racial origin. The development of anaemia or of a transfusion requirement in a patient known to have thalassaemia trait should suggest additional folate or Cbl deficiency.

Rarely Cbl neuropathy may present in the absence of macrocytosis and even with a normoblastic marrow. Presumably such a patient has a substantial dietary folate intake which has maintained normoblastic haemopoiesis.

When the normal MCV is set on the basis of excluding plasma in the haematocrit, the range in healthy adults is 80–90 fl and in megaloblastic anaemia up to about 135 fl. Increases in the MCV up to 95 fl are so commonplace that investigation should normally be undertaken at an MCV above 95 fl.

White blood cells   A fall in the total white blood cell (WBC) count occurs with more severe anaemia. Generally when the red cell count is below 2 × 10^6/μl the total WBC count is below 3 × 10^3/μl.

Platelets   More severe anaemia is accompanied by a reduced platelet

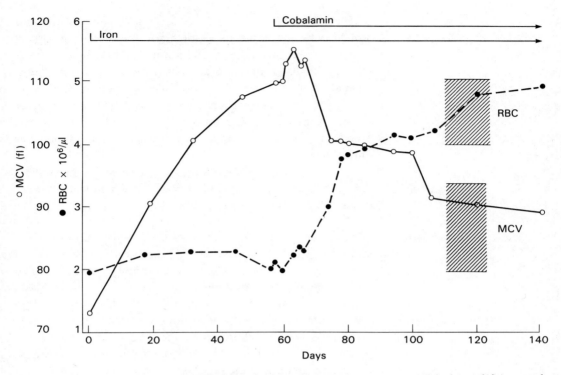

Fig. 2.5 The haematological changes in a patient with both iron deficiency and Cbl deficiency both due to a strict vegetarian diet in a Hindu Indian. Microcytosis was present initially with an MCV of 73 fl and a red cell count of $1.9 \times 10^6/\mu l$. On oral iron there was little change in the red cell count but a striking increase in the MCV to 110 fl. The marrow was megaloblastic at this time and Cbl therapy was followed by a rise of the red cell count and fall of the MCV to normal. The hatched areas indicate the normal range.

count and this is generally below $100 \times 10^3/\mu l$ when the red cell count is below $2 \times 10^6/\mu l$.

Peripheral blood film   In patients with little anaemia uniform macrocytosis is present. Much is made in the literature of oval macrocytes in distinguishing the macrocytosis of megaloblastic patients. Most films do not show this and it is more evident in more severe anaemia with a significant degree of anisocytosis and poikilocytosis. Some films show much red cell fragmentation and such patients may have a relatively lower MCV. In severe cases circulating megaloblasts may be present.

The white cells are essentially normal in early cases. As anaemia develops there is an increase in neutrophils with five or more lobes in the nucleus. It is unusual to have more than 3% of neutrophils with five lobes in normal blood.

It is generally not possible to distinguish between Cbl and folate deficiency from blood or marrow examination. However, the presence of features indicating loss of splenic function in the blood film — target cells, Howell–Jolly bodies, unusually large numbers of erythroblasts and red cell fragments — may suggest either coeliac disease with splenic atrophy or gastrectomy with splenectomy. The megaloblastic anaemia in the former is always due to folate deficiency, and in the latter most likely to Cbl deficiency.

In other cases the blood film is that of a severe haemolytic anaemia or chronic myelofibrosis in which megaloblastosis due to folate deficiency has supervened.

Bone marrow   The essential features have been described in the introduction. Megaloblastosis may be concealed completely by severe iron deficiency or more usually be modified by iron deficiency or accompanying thalassaemia trait. In all cases megaloblasts are best recognized in polychromatic erythroblasts in the edges of the film where material is thinly spread. The diagnostic feature is the fine character of the nuclear chromatin. In a normoblast relatively large areas of chromatin are separated by a few clefts. In a megaloblast the chromatin appears as if a series of small holes have been punched through it with a pin. With a little experience, in properly stained and fixed material, recognition of megaloblasts is relatively easy.

The inexperienced enthusiast tends to be carried away and starts to see megaloblasts in too many marrows. Very minor and uncertain changes must be ignored. Even when the haemoglobin concentration is 17 g/dl, if the macrocytosis is due to true Cbl or folate deficiency, the recognition of megaloblasts is not difficult. If it is difficult, call it normoblastic and you will almost always be right. Do not be biased by information that the Cbl or folate level is low.

The diagnosis of megaloblastosis is a morphological one based on the blood count and the appearance of blood and marrow spreads. If it is intended to make a firm diagnosis of megaloblastosis then a marrow is essential in order to distinguish patients having one of the disorders associated with normoblastic macrocytosis from those with significant Cbl or folate deficiency. This has to be done at the start of an investigation and not after a series of Cbl absorption tests have served to muddy the waters and remove evidence of Cbl deficiency. All too often this is not appreciated by physicians without a specific interest in blood disorders.

Megaloblastosis in other tissues

The changes that occur in replicating cells other than those in marrow are in essence no different from those present in erythroblasts. The cell is larger than normal, the nuclear diameter is larger and in some cells such as those in the buccal mucosa, the nuclear pattern shows a finer meshwork not unlike that of the megaloblast. Such changes have been demonstrated in the buccal mucosa, tongue, nasal mucosa, urinary tract, vagina, cervix uteri, conjunctiva and stomach. In the respiratory system macrophages from the lung of patients with pernicious anaemia are twice the normal size and the bronchial epithelium is abnormal. Enterocytes lining the jejunum obtained by biopsy show enlarged nuclei and overall enlargement of the cell. Transformed lymphocytes from patients with megaloblastic anaemia were larger than normal and were reported to show a more finely open chromatic pattern than controls. These changes have been reviewed [7].

In all cases these changes return to normal after appropriate therapy. These changes may prove puzzling in cytological examination of material from the sputum and uterine cervical smear and have caused confusion because they may be similar to changes seen in pre-malignant lesions.

Suggestions have been made that epithelial changes can be the result of localized folate deficiency, for example in bronchial epithelium in smokers [8]. Since nutrients come via the circulation the only reason for localized changes would be a rapid rate of cell division and hence a high folate requirement but it would be surprising if local megaloblastosis were not accompanied by similar changes in marrow cells.

The deoxyuridine suppression test

The deoxyuridine (dU) suppression test is abnormal in virtually all patients with megaloblastosis and hence is a measure of this state of haemopoiesis [9–10]. It depends on demonstrating an impairment in the synthesis of thymidine by marrow cells which require intact Cbl and folate pathways. Thymidine is available to the dividing cell from two sources, by synthesis and by re-utilizing preformed thymidine which is termed the salvage pathway.

A suspension of bone marrow cells is prepared and an aliquot is incubated with deoxyuridine monophosphate which is a precursor of thymidine. The deoxyuridine is methylated to thymidine by accepting a 1-carbon unit from methylenetetrahydrofolate. The thymidine is then incorporated into DNA (Fig. 2.6). After a short incubation period during which the cell methylates its deoxyuridine, [^{3}H]-labelled thymidine

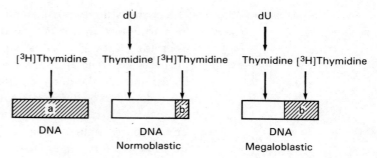

Fig. 2.6 A suspension of bone marrow cells is prepared. One aliquot is incubated with [³H]thymidine. Further aliquots are incubated with deoxyuridine (dU) alone as well as with dU plus Cbl and dU + folinic acid. After 15 min [³H]thymidine is added to these incubation mixtures. DNA is extracted and [³H] activity counted. Marrow cells take up dU, convert it into thymidine and incorporate this into DNA. Any requirement for thymidine not met by synthesis from dU is met by using pre-formed [³H]thymidine. The result is expressed as

$$\frac{\text{Counts in dU sample } (\equiv b)}{\text{Counts without dU } (\equiv a)} \times 100\%.$$

Normally this is less than 10% and with megaloblastic marrows more than 10% (see Table 2.1).

is added and any residual requirement for thymidine not met by synthesis, is met by utilizing [³H]thymidine by the salvage pathway. After this DNA is extracted and the preparation counted for [³H]activity. A 100% value is obtained by incubating an aliquot of marrow with [³H]thymidine alone. With a normoblastic marrow, less than 10% of the labelled thymidine is incorporated into DNA.

In megaloblastic anaemia, because of an impairment of either Cbl or folate metabolism, the synthetic pathway is less effective in methylating deoxyuridine and hence more than 10% of the labelled thymidine appears in DNA. Such a result can range from 10 to 60%. Examples are shown in Table 2.1.

The usefulness of the test can be extended by incubating further aliquots of the marrow cell suspension with Cbl or folate as well as deoxyuridine. In Cbl deficiency there is partial correction of the defect when Cbl is added.

Formyltetrahydrofolate (folinic acid, leucovorin) produces a full correction in both Cbl and folate deficiency. Thus the nature of the deficiency causing megaloblastosis can be determined as well.

Occasionally abnormal results have been obtained in apparently simple iron deficiency, epileptics taking anticonvulsant drugs and in protein–calorie malnutrition [11]. The

Table 2.1 Results in the deoxyuridine (dU) suppression test expressed as

$$\frac{\text{Counts }[^3\text{H}]\text{ in DNA in marrow with dU}}{\text{Counts }[^3\text{H}]\text{ in DNA in marrow without dU}} \times 100\%*$$

Patient	1	2	3
No additive	6.5	18.0	24.0
Cbl added	6.7	14.6	24.6
Folinic acid added	5.9	7.8	6.8
Interpretation	Normal	Cbl deficiency	Folate deficiency

* Normal less than 10%.

author has encountered abnormal results in the dU suppression when the marrow was essentially normoblastic although the patient probably had either Cbl or folate deficiency.

The test is time consuming and its performance may take much of the day. For this reason it has not been widely adopted outside research centres. It has been suggested that a mitogen-stimulated lymphocyte culture is a substitute for marrow cells. This is not the case. Normal replicating lymphocytes rapidly run out of folate so that after 24 hours they start to behave like folate-deficient marrow cells [11].

Clinical biochemistry   A variety of changes accompany megaloblastic anaemia. These are absent in early cases with little anaemia and become more marked in anaemic subjects.

A reduced serum potassium level may be present in anaemic patients (3.2–3.9 mmol/l) and in some series this has been noted in almost half the patients. Red cell potassium was low in 11 out of 18 patients. In a few elderly patients a further fall in serum potassium may occur a few days after giving specific therapy and some have regarded this as an indication for giving potassium supplements.

Icterus may be present in some patients and a larger number, perhaps 30%, have a raised serum bilirubin level. This is related to ineffective haemopoiesis with death of megaloblasts in the marrow. The jaundice is haemolytic in type and the bilirubin falls within hours of giving specific therapy.

There is a small but consistent fall in the gammaglobulin level and IgG immunoglobulins and there is a rise following specific therapy. Neonates with untreated megaloblastic anaemia are unable to mount an immune response, although following treatment, antibodies to antigens administered in the pre-treatment phase all duly appear [12].

Plasma free amino acids are raised and this is accompanied

by aminoaciduria. Amino acids appearing in urine include lysine, taurine, *p*-amino-isobutyric acid, aspartic acid, tyrosine, phenylalanine and leucine. Increased taurine excretion was noted in 44 out of 57 patients. The excretion declines after specific therapy.

Reduced plasma cholesterol [13] as well as lipid levels occur and rise following therapy.

Serum iron increases with severity of anaemia (Fig. 2.7) but the transferrin level tends to be reduced and is about 50% saturated [7]. The mean serum ferritin level in 30 patients was 330 µg/l as compared to 164 µg/l in controls. Except in pregnancy, postgastrectomy and coeliac disease iron stores are adequate and usually increased.

The activity of most enzymes that have been measured in plasma and red cells are increased, sometimes strikingly so. The explanation for this is not clear, but as impaired Cbl/folate function may lead to defective transmethylation, it is tempting to speculate that the hypomethylation of cytosine residues in DNA activates a large number of genes which in turn increase the concentration of enzymes they produce [434]. The best studied is lactic acid dehydrogenase (LDH) where values exceeding 10 000 units/ml/min are not uncommon in untreated megaloblastic anaemia. The mean level in 16 patients was 3800 units/ml/min as compared to 260 units/ml/min in controls [14]. Other enzymes showing increased activity include λ-hydroxybutyrate dehydrogenase, glucose-6-phosphate dehy-

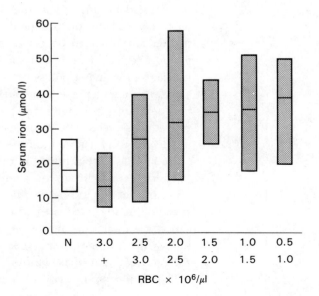

Fig. 2.7 Mean and range of serum iron concentration in untreated pernicious anaemia in relation to the red cell count.

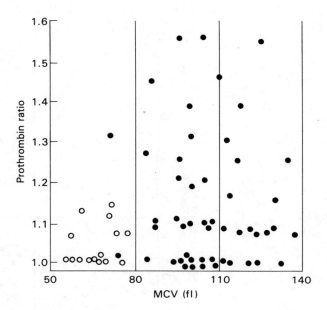

Fig. 2.8 Prothrombin ratio in patients with megaloblastic anaemia (●) and in iron-deficiency anaemia (○) with comparable haemoglobin levels. (Unpublished data, Y. Stirling.)

drogenase, malic dehydrogenase, aldolase, etc. These levels decline within a few days of treatment.

Similarly red cell enzymes show increased activity. These include enzymes of the Embden–Myerhof pathway, methaemoglobin reductase, catalase, carbonic anhydrase, etc. as well as enzymes concerned with pyrimidine synthesis. Thymidine kinase measured in lymphocytes had six times the activity in megalobastic patients as in controls [15]. The activity of 2,3-diphosphoglycerate (2,3-DPG) also increases in megaloblastic anaemia as a compensation for anaemia and the effect is to decrease the affinity of haemoglobin for oxygen. This shifts the oxygen dissociation curve to the right (increases P50) and so makes oxygen more readily available to tissues. This results in an increase in tissue oxygen supply of about 30% in a patient with 7.5 g/dl of haemoglobin.

Severe megaloblastic anaemia may be associated with a prolonged prothrombin time (Fig. 2.8), low fibrinogen levels and slightly prolonged thrombin time. Bruising can be due to severe thrombocytopenia but in some there is evidence of disseminated intravascular coagulation with low fibrinogen, increased fibrin-degradation products and fibrin monomers.

Intestinal malabsorption is present in about one-third of patients with megaloblastic anaemia and abnormal tests disappear after therapy. Thirty-seven out of 124 patients with

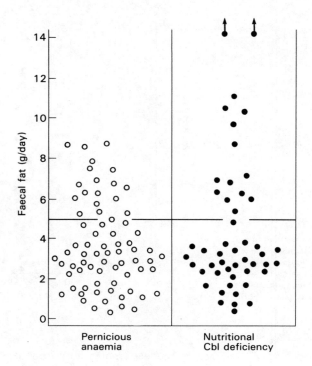

Fig. 2.9 Daily faecal fat excretion in untreated patients with megaloblastic anaemia on a 100 g fat intake.

megaloblastic anaemia excreted more than 5 g fat a day on a 100 g fat intake (Fig. 2.9) [16]. Twenty-two out of 57 patients had impaired xylose absorption. A transient impairment of absorption of Cbl linked to intrinsic factor may be present, and this as well as other evidence of malabsorption, are corrected after specific therapy.

Ferrokinetics, ineffective haemopoiesis and red cell life span

The way labelled iron is handled before and after treatment in megaloblastic anaemia illustrates the defects in erythropoiesis.

^{59}Fe given intravenously to a patient with well-established megaloblastic anaemia is cleared from plasma more rapidly than normal. This is due to uptake by an active marrow. However, the amount of ^{59}Fe incorporated into red cells during the next 2 weeks is reduced (Fig. 2.10). Thus normally between 60 and 100% of ^{59}Fe is incorporated into red cells whereas in pernicious anaemia this ranges from very small amounts to a maximum of 45% of the dose.

The plasma iron turnover is an index of erythropoiesis and averages about 27 mg/day in normal subjects. This is markedly increased in megaloblastic anaemia ranging from 59 to 145 mg/day. The discrepancy between the high iron turnover and

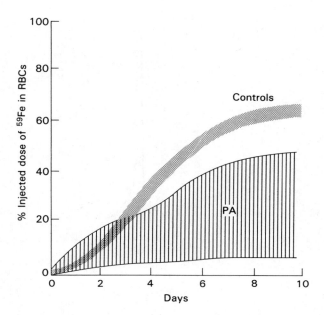

Fig. 2.10 ^{59}Fe is given intravenously and its incorporation into red cells followed over 10 days. In patients with untreated pernicious anaemia iron incorporation is less than that found in controls.

the poor utilization of iron for red cell formation is due to markedly ineffective haemopoiesis with considerable death of cells in the marrow.

Ineffective haemopoiesis can be quantitated in a number of ways and in particular by the faecal excretion of ^{15}N-glycine (Fig. 2.11). Glycine is incorporated into haem in the early erythroblast. Normally about one in ten erythroblasts fail to mature and the haem in these cells is excreted as stercobilin. Thus when ^{15}N-glycine is used to label haem, about 11% of the label is excreted in the first 8 days and the remaining 89% at about 100 days at the end of the life span of the red cells. In megaloblastic anaemia, because of considerable intramedullary death of cells that have failed to mature, up to 40% of the label is excreted 5–12 days after giving the label.

Ineffective erythropoiesis can also be demonstrated by measuring [^{3}H]thymidine incorporation into erythroblasts. In megaloblastic anaemia a high proportion of cells are unable to complete DNA synthesis with values between $2n$ and $4n$ ($2n$ being the DNA content of a diploid cell). Such cells presumably die in the marrow.

Surface counting in megaloblastic anaemia shows that a dose of ^{59}Fe accumulates initially in marrow and liver but thereafter is shifted into the liver rather than into red cells.

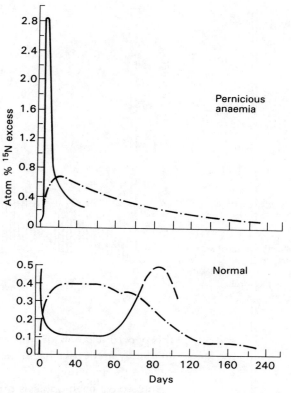

Fig. 2.11 [^{15}N]glycine is incorporated into haem. About 10% is excreted as stercobilin in faeces within the first 10 days and this is the normal wastage among developing erythroblasts. The rest of the [^{15}N]glycine is incorporated into haem mainly into a cohort of red blood cells and this appears in faeces as stercobilin at the end of the red cell life span. This is shown in the lower portion of the figure with rise of [^{15}N] in haem in the first 10 days, a plateau and then its disappearance from blood as this cohort reaches the end of its life span.

By contrast in pernicious anaemia there is markedly increased wastage with about 40% of haem being lost in the early days due to ineffective haemopoiesis. Thereafter there is a steady decline in the [^{15}N] haem in blood due to random destruction of red cells because of the haemolytic component of the anaemia. ——— Stercobilin, · ——— · haem.

Treatment causes a remarkable reversal of all these phenomena. There is an abrupt fall in serum iron and serum ferritin. The clearance of iron becomes even more rapid. Labelled iron leaves marrow and liver and appears in blood in new red blood cells (Fig. 2.12). Ineffective haemopoiesis rapidly becomes effective and serum bilirubin falls within hours (Fig. 2.13).

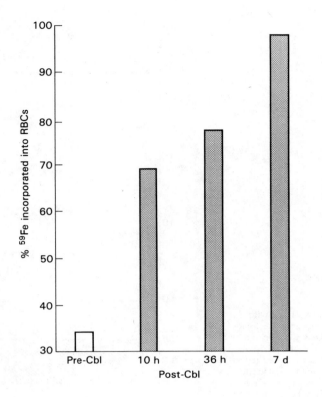

Fig. 2.12 The incorporation of ^{59}Fe into red cells was only 34% of the dose before Cbl treatment in pernicious anaemia. Within 10 hours of Cbl it was 68%, at 36 hours 74% and after 7 days 96%. [104].

Life span of macrocytes

Normal red blood cells survive for about 110 days in the circulation. In well-developed megaloblastic anaemia, red cell survival is shortened significantly (from 28 to 75 days). However, the survival of normal red cells transfused to a patient with untreated megaloblastic anaemia is similarly shortened indicating the presence of an extracorpuscular factor. The nature of this factor is not understood. Whatever its nature, in pernicious anaemia it disappears 9 days after an injection of Cbl [17]. Haptoglobins are usually absent in untreated megaloblastic anaemia providing further evidence of the reduction in red cell life span.

Chromosomes

The metaphases obtained from marrow in patients with megaloblastic anaemia are abnormal. The abnormalities consist of breakages which may involve any chromosome and show themselves as acentric fragments, gaps or breaks. Incomplete contraction in metaphase is striking in about 25% of marrows [18].

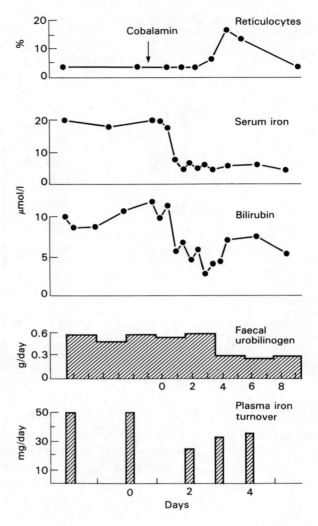

Fig. 2.13 This patient with pernicious anaemia was treated with Cbl. This was followed by a reticulocytosis, and fall in the serum iron as iron is shifted to the marrow. There is a fall in the serum bilirubin as excessive wastage of erythroblasts in the marrow ceases and this is the explanation for the fall in faecal urobilinogen which is derived from haem breakdown. Plasma iron turnover which is increased from 27 mg/day to between 59 and 145 mg/day in untreated pernicious anaemia due to ineffectual haemopoiesis, declines.

Elongation of individual chromosomes is a significant feature in culture and the increase may be about 25% as compared to normal chromosomes. All the abnormalities disappear after specific treatment. These defects may be related to impaired methylation of DNA cytosine residues. The state of methylation of cytosine has been shown to have profound effects on orientation and coiling of plasmid DNA [19].

Chapter 3   Normal cobalamin metabolism

Structure   Cobalamin (Fig. 3.1) is made up of four pyrrole rings (A–D). Three are joined by intervening carbon units and the last pair by a direct link. This ring is the corrin nucleus. In Cbl the four pyrroles have a cobalt atom at the centre to which they are all joined.

A nucleotide (5,6-dimethylbenziminazole) is also attached to the central cobalt atom as well as to one of the pyrrole rings by a sugar (ribofuranose) and a chain called amino-2-propanol.

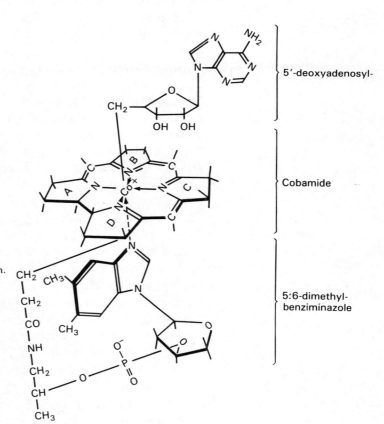

Fig. 3.1 Deoxyadenosylcobalamin. The four pyrrole rings are numbered A, B, C and D and they are joined by a carbon other than rings A and D which are joined directly. A nucleotide (benziminazole) is set at right angles to the plane of the corrin nucleus. The nucleotide as well as each of the four pyrrole rings are also attached to cobalt at the centre of cobamide. In adoCbl deoxyadenosine is also linked to the Co atom.

23

The attachment of the nucleotide to the cobalt is variable and in some states the nucleotide is free (termed base-off position).

Not only is the cobalt attached to the four pyrrole rings and to benziminazole but it has a further valency that carries a ligand — either methyl, deoxyadenosyl or hydroxo and, in an abnormal situation, either cyano or sulphito. The first three are the physiological analogues.

The cobalt atom exists in a variable state of oxidation — fully reduced it is termed Cob(I)alamin or B_{12s} as in the form required for synthesis of methionine, partially oxidized is Cob(II)alamin or B_{12r} and fully oxidized Cob(III)alamin or B_{12}. Cob(I)alamin reacts with the anaesthetic gas, nitrous oxide (N_2O) which cleaves the N_2O molecule and which oxidizes the Cbl to a biologically inactive form. Prolonged N_2O inhalation in man produces fatal megaloblastic anaemia and intermittent inhalation cobalamin neuropathy [20–22].

Cobalamin reductases are present in the cells of both the cytosol and mitochondria. They affect cob(I)alamin formation and their absence gives rise to rare inherited methylmalonic acidurias.

Biochemical role

In mammals only two roles have been identified for cobalamin: the *de novo* synthesis of methionine and the conversion of methylmalonic acid to succinic acid. This somewhat limited repertoire belies the central role that Cbl plays in maintaining normal folate metabolism. Indeed, it is still difficult to reconcile the limited biochemical role of Cbl with the diverse effects on haemopoiesis and the central nervous system (CNS) in man caused by its deficiency.

Homocysteine methyltransferase

Both folate and Cbl are required for the addition of a methyl group to homocysteine to form methionine (Fig. 3.2). The single carbon unit from serine or formate is transferred to reduced folate (tetrahydrofolate). The single carbon is further reduced to the $-CH_3$ or methyl form (5-methyltetrahydrofolate). The enzyme, homocysteine methyltransferase (or methionine synthetase), transfers the methyl to Cbl to yield methylcobalamin and, finally, the methyl is passed to homocysteine to form methionine (Fig. 3.3). Methionine in turn is converted to S-adenosylmethionine which is the major source of methyl groups in transmethylation reactions. The transfer of the methyl group from S-adenosylmethionine results in the formation of S-adenosylhomocysteine which after removal of adenosine is once again remethylated to methionine

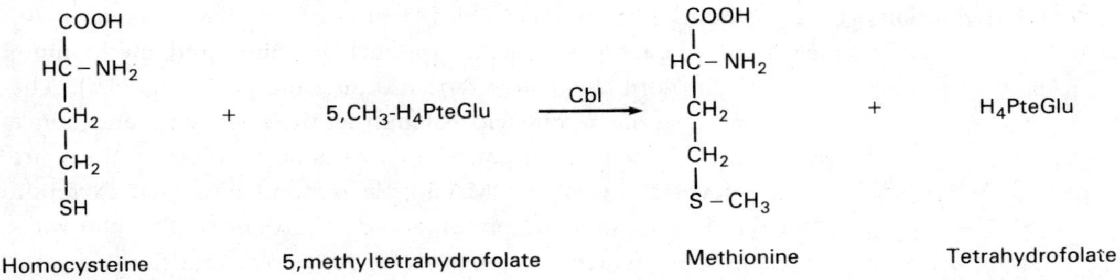

COOH   COOH

HC – NH₂   HC – NH₂

CH₂   +   5,CH₃-H₄PteGlu ──Cbl──→   CH₂   +   H₄PteGlu

CH₂   CH₂

SH   S – CH₃

Homocysteine   5,methyltetrahydrofolate   Methionine   Tetrahydrofolate

Fig. 3.2 The enzyme methionine synthetase of which Cbl is a coenzyme, transfers the methyl group from methyltetrahydrofolate to homocysteine in the *de novo* synthesis of methionine.

(Fig. 3.4). In megaloblastic anaemia where there is impairment of this pathway, plasma homocysteine levels are elevated [23].

The reaction is of particular interest because both folate and Cbl coenzymes are concerned and this relationship has proved to be central to our understanding of cobalamin–folate interrelations.

Fig. 3.3 A single carbon unit either as formate (–CHO) or methylene (–CH₂–) on tetrahydrofolate is reduced to methyl(–CH₃) and transferred to cobalamin and then to homocysteine. In this reaction the Cbl is the coenzyme of methionine synthetase.

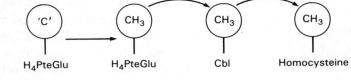

'C'   CH₃   CH₃   CH₃

H₄PteGlu   H₄PteGlu   Cbl   Homocysteine

Formyl- or methylene-   5,methyl-   Methyl-   Methionine
tetrahydrofolate   tetrahydrofolate cobalamin

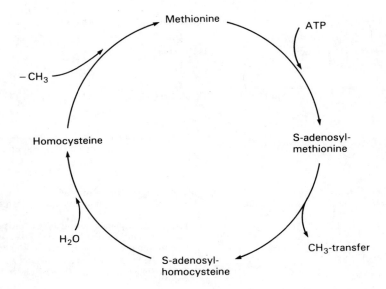

Methionine

ATP

– CH₃

S-adenosyl-
methionine

Homocysteine

CH₃-transfer

H₂O

S-adenosyl-
homocysteine

Fig. 3.4 About half the methionine in man is converted to S-adenosylmethionine which is the major transmethylating agent. In turn it is converted to S-adenosyls homocysteine. This compound is toxic and rapidly loses its adenine to become homocysteine.

Methylmalonyl-CoA
mutase

Methylmalonic acid (MMA) arises from the metabolism of propionic acid, leucine, isoleucine, valine and methionine. It is normally converted into succinic acid (Fig. 3.5). The mutase has adenosylcobalamin as the coenzyme and hence the pathway is impaired in Cbl deficiency when there are elevated levels of MMA in plasma and increased excretion in urine. In addition inherited disorders of the pathways which involve a racemase enzyme converting the D enantiomorph of MMA to the L enantiomorph and reductases required to process Cbl in the cell may be abnormal, and may produce methylmalonylaciduria.

Dietary cobalamin

The source of cobalamin is microbial synthesis. It is totally absent from the plant kingdom and a strict vegetarian diet does not contain Cbl other than that which may arise from bacterial contamination. Herbivorous animals have a rich Cbl-producing microbial flora in the foregut which is their source of Cbl. Fruit bats inadvertently consume insects on the surface of fruit which provide them with Cbl. Fruit bats fed washed fruit die of Cbl deficiency in about 9 months.

Cbl is present in all foodstuffs of animal origin including dairy produce, fish, poultry and meat. Liver is a very rich source. It is a stable compound resisting cooking and is only destroyed in very alkaline conditions (pH 12).

A mixed diet supplies about 5 µg Cbl daily [24]. A vegetarian diet contains less than 0.5 µg. The daily Cbl require-

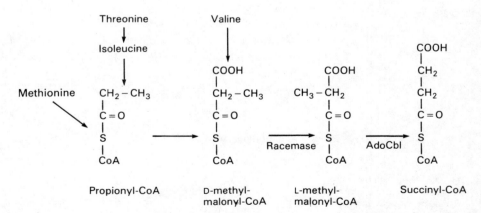

Fig. 3.5 Methylmalonic acid arises from propionate metabolism via threonine, isoleucine and methionine or via valine. A racemase converts D-methylmalonic acid to L-methylmalonic acid which is metabolized to succinate. The latter enters the Krebs cycle. Methylmalonic acid can accumulate when there is absence of a functioning racemase enzyme or absence of adenosylcobalamin.

ment has been deduced largely from studies on loss of Cbl from the body in adults measuring either the Cbl content of urine and faeces or the loss of whole-body radioactivity after a dose of [^{60}Co]Cbl. This figure is of the order of 1–3 μg daily [7] in subjects consuming a mixed diet. It is likely that the minimum requirement to maintain health is less than this and is of the order of 1.0 μg daily.

Tissue cobalamin

The total body pool of Cbl in those taking mixed diets ranges from 2.5 to 5 mg. On the basis of a 3 mg pool and a daily requirement of 1 μg, Cbl stores should suffice for 3000 days. The highest concentration of Cbl in man and other species is in liver which contains about 1 μg Cbl per g of liver and holds about 50% of total body Cbl. Muscle (8.6%), marrow (4.4%) and gut (4.5%) also have significant amounts of Cbl [7].

In the cell Cbl is found in the cytosol as methylCbl and in mitochondria as adenosylCbl. In these two sites the Cbl is the coenzyme for methionine synthetase in cytosol and for methylmalonyl-CoA mutase in mitochondria. AdenosylCbl is the predominant analogue in tissues in man. Liver contains 61% deoxyadenosylCbl, 38% hydroxoCbl and 1% methylCbl but other tissues may have between 10 and 30% methylCbl. Plasma contains 65% methylCbl [25] and milk 58%.

Absorption and transport of cobalamin

Cobalamin is a large hydrophilic molecule (molecular weight (MW) 1355 daltons) and specialized mechanisms have evolved to transport it from the diet into the enterocyte and out of the enterocyte into plasma and into tissue cells. Free Cbl does not exist in mammals other than during the few hours following a large parenteral injection of Cbl. Two important transport proteins are involved and a third Cbl-binding protein is present in all tissues and secretions for which no specific role has been identified.

Intrinsic factor (IF)

IF is a glycoprotein (MW 45 000 daltons) that is secreted by the gastric-parietal cell in man. Stimulants which increase hydrochloric acid production also increase the output of IF. Maximum secretion accompanies a meal. The additional IF secretion on continuous stimulation, for example, with gastrin and its analogues, consists of a rapid initial phase due to the release of stored IF from the parietal cell followed by a steady output above baseline levels due to new synthesis of IF. The amount of IF available far exceeds the amount of Cbl requiring absorption. A unit of IF is defined as the amount binding 1 ng Cbl. Five hundred IF units produce maximum absorption of an oral dose of 1 µg Cbl. [26]. On the other hand the IF output over 24 hours may exceed 100 000 ng units. IF is heat labile and is destroyed by proteolytic enzymes present in the gastrointestinal (GI) tract. At neutral pH it is stable for many months in the frozen state.

Transcobalamin II (TCII)   TCII is the prime transporter of Cbl. In the absence of a functional TCII severe megaloblastic anaemia ensues. It is a polypeptide (MW 38 000 daltons) which is secreted by the liver, macrophages, ileal cells, endothelial cells [27] and perhaps many other cells as well. It is excreted into plasma at a steady rate and following a large injection of Cbl which exceeds the capacity of Cbl-binding proteins in plasma, free TCII reaccumulates within minutes of the disappearance of free Cbl from plasma. The Cbl binding capacity of plasma is due largely to its TCII content. This may be expressed in terms of the amount of Cbl bound per unit plasma. One ml plasma contains enough TCII to bind about 600 pg Cbl. Cell surfaces contain receptors for TCII–Cbl complex which is then internalized by pinocytosis so releasing Cbl into the cell. The half-life of the TCII–Cbl complex in plasma in man is about 60 min. TCII is composed of several isoproteins which vary in their electrophoretic mobility. These patterns are inherited [28]. The gene for TCII is on chromosome 22.

R-binders   All body fluids including plasma contain a Cbl-binding glycoprotein which on electrophoresis moves more rapidly than TCII, hence the name rapid or R-binder. Other terms such as TCI and haptocorrin have been given to this glycoprotein but the term R-binder will be used in this text. R-binders in all body fluids have the same protein moiety but differences in carbohydrate content have been reported for R-binder from saliva, plasma and leucocytes. An R-binder in the specific granules of neutrophil leucocytes has been termed TCIII. The half-life of Cbl on R-binder in man is about 9 days. Because of this long half-life most of the Cbl in plasma is that bound to R-binder. The free R-binder of plasma is able to bind about 40 pg Cbl. No specific role has been assigned to R-binder. One hypothesis is that it mops up free Cbl which may be released following tissue destruction as may occur in sites of inflammation. The R-binder–Cbl complex is cleared by the liver.

More recently an attempt has been made to correlate lack of R-binder with unusual neurological syndromes [29].

Intestinal phase of cobalamin absorption

The function of IF is to bind to Cbl. This it does extremely rapidly and in a stoichiometric manner. IF–Cbl, unlike free IF, is relatively resistant to proteolytic digestion as it needs to be since the site of absorption of Cbl is in the distal ileum. Dietary Cbl is in the form of protein-bound Cbl. Peptic digestion releases Cbl as a free form. Although the Cbl-binding proteins in gastric juice consist of 90% IF and only 10% R-binder, the acid pH appears to favour Cbl binding to R-binder. Thus initially some 50% of the Cbl is IF-bound and 50% R-binder bound. In the jejunum pancreatic proteolytic enzymes cleave the R-binder and release Cbl to bind to free IF.

The IF–Cbl complex traverses the small gut. In the ileum specific receptors for the complex are present on the surface of ileal enterocytes (Fig. 3.6). The ileal receptor for IF–Cbl is synthesized in the villus crypt and moves up the villus into the microvillus pits in the villus tip cells [30]. The receptor is a membrane protein consisting of two subunits: a smaller alpha unit which binds the IF–Cbl complex very tightly and a larger beta unit which traverses the cell membrane. In the pig the MW of the two units exceed 200 000 daltons. Calcium ions and a neutral pH are required for receptor binding of IF–Cbl. Several receptors cluster together to form hexagons or pentagons, hence the high MW found on primary isolation of these receptors [31]. After the attachment of IF–Cbl to the receptor, events are uncertain. Cbl entering portal blood does so attached to TCII [32]. Thus IF dose not enter portal blood. Whether IF separates from Cbl at the receptor, or whether the complex is internalized in the enterocyte before separation, has not been established.

Fig. 3.6 Cobalamin and IF link in a stoichiometric manner and the complex is taken up by specific receptors in enterocytes at the tips of ileal villi. Cbl separates from IF and a Cbl– transcobalamin II (TCII) complex enters portal blood.

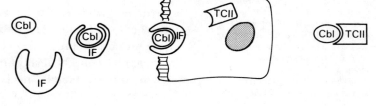

Gut lumen   Ileal enterocyte   Portal blood

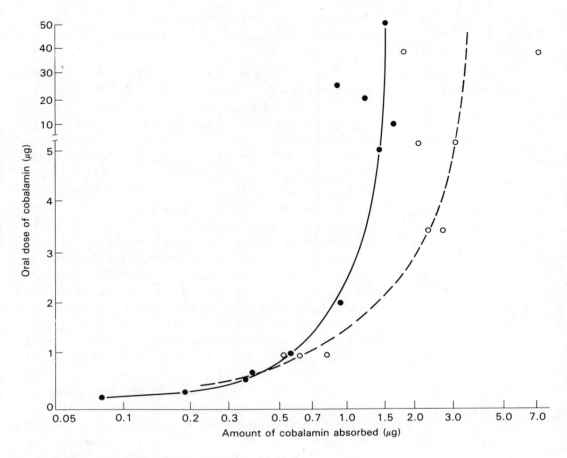

Fig. 3.7 There is a limit to the amount of cobalamin that is absorbed from a single dose. Varying oral doses of labelled Cbl in aqueous solution were given to volunteers and the mean amount absorbed at each dose level is shown (●). This indicates a maximum absorption of about 1.5 µg. Labelled food Cbl was prepared by giving $^{60}CoCl_2$ to lambs and ultimately obtaining meat and liver with a ^{60}Co-label in Cbl. When fed to volunteers (○) a similar limitation to absorption was found as with aqueous Cbl [33]. Too few observations are available to conclude that native Cbl is better absorbed than an aqueous solution of Cbl although the diagram suggests that this may be so.

The amount of Cbl that can be absorbed from a single oral dose is limited to a maximum of about 1.5–2 µg (Fig. 3.7). The likely reason is limitation in the numbers of ileal receptors. A second dose of Cbl given 3 hours later is absorbed normally. Further, food Cbl such as that present in lamb is absorbed in the same way and in the same amount as aqueous Cbl [33]. It has been reported that Cbl is absorbed badly when given with egg white [34] and other substances such as chick serum which binds Cbl very avidly, may make the Cbl unavailable for absorption.

The final phase in Cbl absorption is passage out of the ileal enterocyte to portal blood. This is achieved by Cbl linking in the enterocyte to TCII and the resulting TCII–Cbl complex entering the blood. In man the peak blood level after an oral dose of Cbl is reached after 8–12 hours. The events responsible for this lag have not been resolved although it is assumed to be related to separation of Cbl from IF or perhaps synthesis of TCII.

The role of Transcobalamin II

Virtually all cells have specific receptors for TCII to which TCII–Cbl attaches. Entry of Cbl into the cell is by receptor-mediated endocytosis (Fig. 3.8). It is probable that TCII is degraded after internalization. During Cbl absorption the bulk of the Cbl is delivered to the liver and hepatic radioactivity after a dose of Cbl has been used as a test of Cbl absorption.

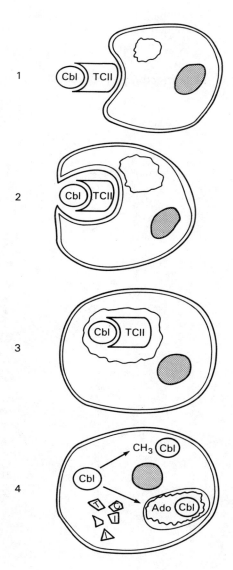

Fig. 3.8 The Cbl–transcobalamin complex is taken up by specific receptors on the cell surface (1) and internalized by endocytosis (2). A secondary lysosome is formed (3). TCII is probably degraded and Cbl converted to a coenzyme in cytosol (methylCbl) or in mitochondria (adoCbl) (4).

Enterohepatic circulation

Cbl undergoes an enterohepatic circulation, the Cbl content of bile ranging from 1000 to 11000 pg/ml. IF is required to reabsorb the Cbl [7].

Cobalamin level in man

The normal level of Cbl in plasma and serum is 170–1000 pg/ml. The bulk is carried in the alpha globulin region on R-binder and about 10% is carried on TCII which is located in the beta globulin region.

Cbl may be measured by microbiological assay usually with *Lactobacillus leichmannii* or *Euglena gracilis* as test organisms. It may also be measured by saturation analysis techniques which assess the dilution of a standard amount of labelled Cbl by the native Cbl of plasma using purified IF as the binding agent in the test. All these methods, when performed correctly, give essentially the same results.

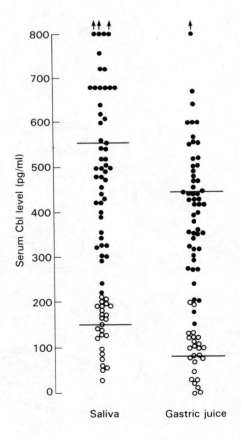

Fig. 3.9 The serum Cbl level has been assayed in healthy controls (●) and in patients with untreated pernicious anaemia (○) using isotopically labelled Cbl in a saturation analysis assay. On the right are results when gastric juice containing almost 99% IF as the Cbl binder was used and on the left the results when saliva which contains only R-binder, was used. Results are higher when the R-binder is used in the assay because R-binder attaches to Cbl analogues not detected by IF. Both assays are able to differentiate sera from controls and pernicious anaemia patients, although a few controls overlapped the pernicious anaemia group. The horizontal line is the mean Cbl level in each group.

If in carrying out a saturation analysis assay, an R-binder is used as the binding agent (instead of IF), further Cbl analogues are detected in all sera often in about equal amounts to that found with an IF assay (Fig. 3.9). The identity of these Cbl analogues has caused considerable interest. The probability is that they are physiological products of Cbl metabolism since they are present in cord blood and their concentration declines with the total Cbl level. It has not been possible to separate these analogues from microbiologically-active Cbls by conventional means. On a small scale, however, polyacrylamide beads coated with human IF have been used to adsorb out all microbiological active Cbls leaving behind these Cbl analogues [35]. Although it has been conjectured that these analogues are potentially harmful agents absorbed from the diet, this is improbable as the IF absorption mechanism is specific for Cbl. The production of these analogues *in vivo* can be demonstrated in animals exposed to N_2O where their concentration increases substantially in the liver. Perhaps they are a byproduct of the methionine synthetase reaction.

Although there are several reports that the serum Cbl level declines with age, it is usually impossible to exclude situations among the elderly that may lead to reduced Cbl levels. In particular, simple atrophic gastritis can depress Cbl absorption and can be accompanied by a reduced serum Cbl level. It is thus difficult to accept the claim of a reduced Cbl level with age. The lower limit of normal should remain at 170 pg/ml.

Subjects of African origin, be they Caribbean or US negroes, have higher Cbl levels than Caucasians.

Red blood cells have a Cbl content of 85–225 pg/ml of washed packed cells (mean 155).

The Cbl level in CSF is much lower than that in plasma, ranging from about 5 to 60 pg/ml (mean about 20). These low levels are difficult to assay with any degree of confidence.

The Cbl content of human liver ranges from 0.6 to 1.5 µg/g wet liver (mean 1.0 µg) and 0.7–79 ng/mg protein (mean 10 ng).

Chapter 4   Assessment of cobalamin status

There are a number of investigations that are helpful in assessing Cbl status and a diagnosis of Cbl deficiency requires consideration of several of these factors. In particular it is a profound error to equate Cbl deficiency merely with a low serum Cbl level. Many subjects who have low Cbl levels have normal amounts of Cbl in their tissues, for example, in normal pregnancy.

The investigations that may prove helpful in deciding whether a particular patient has Cbl deficiency include the following.

Serum Cbl level.

Deoxyuridine suppression test.

Urinary (and plasma) methylmalonic acid levels.

Gastric secretion and gastric biopsy.

Cbl absorption tests.

Antibodies against IF.

Response to Cbl therapy.

Serum Cbl levels

Samples for Cbl assay must be collected before any specific therapy is given as it may take months before the Cbl level will return to the pre-injection level. Such a dose of Cbl may also remove all other evidence of deficiency in the marrow and elsewhere.

All patients with Cbl deficiency must have a low Cbl level, that is, below 170 pg/ml. The very rare exception are a few patients with myeloproliferative disorders who have extremely high Cbl levels with extremely high R-binder levels in plasma. In such patients superimposed Cbl deficiency will bring down their previously very high Cbl levels (often several 1000 pg/ml) to the conventional normal range.

It is essential to assess laboratory reports in a critical manner. Assay of Cbl levels can be difficult to perform well and poor quality assays abound. It is not unheard of for a normal result to emerge when the true Cbl level is actually low. More often falsely low levels are reported. It is a further reason to ensure that investigations start by establishing that the patient has a megaloblastic marrow.

In general there is a rough correlation between the serum Cbl level and the severity of anaemia — levels in Cbl deficiency range from 20 to 170 pg/ml.

Low serum Cbl levels not associated with clinical Cbl deficiency

Normal subjects

From time to time subjects are seen with Cbl levels below the conventional normal range for which no reason can be established. Such subjects are well clinically and haematologically, have normal Cbl plasma binders and absorb Cbl normally.

Simple atrophic gastritis

Investigations in patients including those with non-ulcer dyspepsia [36] show that a proportion have varying degrees of atrophic gastritis although they are normal haematologically. About 30% of patients with gastric atrophy have low serum Cbl levels [7]. Of these about half also have impaired Cbl absorption. However, follow-up for as long as 30 years indicates that transition into pernicious anaemia is rare [37]. Presumably, although Cbl absorption is reduced, sufficient IF is available to absorb enough Cbl to maintain normoblastic haemopoiesis even if there is not enough in some to maintain a normal serum level.

Vegetarian diet

As Cbl is only present in a vegetarian diet as a result of contamination from bacterial or animal sources, it is not surprising that a very high proportion of such subjects have low serum Cbl levels. Thus among a community of about 15 000 Hindu Indians living in London whose diet is essentially vegetarian or lactovegetarian, 54% of 1000 consecutive blood samples sent to the laboratory showed low Cbl levels. Among this community over a 15-year period 134 cases of megaloblastic anaemia largely due to nutritional Cbl deficiency were seen [16]. Nevertheless the vast majority do not have haematological evidence of Cbl deficiency. No doubt their Cbl intake and Cbl store are well below the levels present in subjects on mixed diets but nevertheless suffice to maintain normal health. There are millions of such persons in India.

Pregnancy

In pregnancy about 5% of healthy women have Cbl levels in the deficiency range as they approach term. In megaloblastic anaemia in pregnancy this rises to 25% of patients. The explanation is the preferential transfer of Cbl from the diet to the placenta and fetus at the expense of maintaining the plasma compartment. As the total Cbl content of a full-term fetus is only about 50 µg the events of one pregnancy cannot have much impact on maternal stores which, in those on mixed diets, are about 3000 µg.

Iron-deficiency anaemia

Occasionally a low serum Cbl is encountered in iron deficiency which returns to normal over a period of months as the iron deficiency is treated. The explanation for this is not clear.

Primary folate deficiency

About one-third of patients with megaloblastic anaemia due to folate deficiency have low serum Cbl levels. These Cbl levels are restored to normal within 7–10 days of starting folate treatment (Fig. 4.1). The explanation is not known. Low Cbl levels may also be seen in epileptics taking anticonvulsant medication.

Comment

It should be evident that a low serum Cbl level alone is of itself inadequate evidence on which to base a diagnosis of Cbl deficiency. Its significance must depend on other accompanying findings. The low Cbl level almost certainly means deficiency when other evidence of pernicious anaemia is found, when associated with impaired Cbl absorption, in strict lifelong vegetarians or when associated with increased levels of methylmalonic acid. On the other hand in patients on a mixed

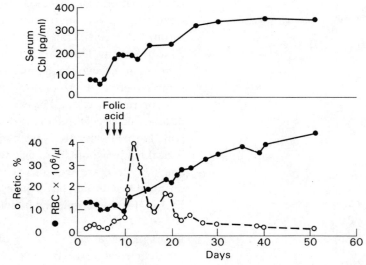

Fig. 4.1 A patient with coeliac disease and a megaloblastic anaemia. The pre-treatment red cell count was $1.3 \times 10^6/\mu l$ and the serum Cbl level 75 pg/ml. Three injections of folic acid, each 15 mg, were given. There was a optimal reticulocyte response reaching 40% on day 6 and a satisfactory rise in red cell count. The serum cobalamin level rose from a base line of 75 pg/ml to 180 pg/ml 3 days after treatment and rose steadily to a plateau.

Table 4.1 The frequency of
low serum cobalamin levels
in disorders associated with
a megaloblastic anaemia

Disorder	Percentage of patients having a low serum Cbl level
Pernicious anaemia	100
Total gastrectomy	100
Partial gastrectomy	15
Adult coeliac disease	25–40
Childhood coeliac disease	0
Abnormal gut flora	85
Crohn's disease	60
Normal pregnancy	14–28
Megaloblastic anaemia in pregnancy	30–44
Anticonvulsant-treated patients	2
Anticonvulsants with megaloblastic anaemia	35
Tropical sprue	80–95
Lactovegetarians	50–75
Fish tapeworm carriers	75
Primary folate deficiency with megaloblastic anaemia	31

diet, normal Cbl absorption should rule out Cbl deficiency. The frequency of low serum cobalamin levels in different situations is shown in Table 4.1.

The deoxyuridine suppression test

This test, carried out on a suspension of marrow cells taken at the time of an aspiration to determine morphology, is particularly useful in potentially difficult cases. The details have been set out on p. 13. An abnormal result, that is greater that 10% uptake of [^{3}H]thymidine, occurs with megaloblastic marrows. The addition of Cbl produces partial correction in marrows from Cbl-deficient patients but no change in those who are folate deficient. Folates, particularly 5-formyltetrahydrofolate, produce full correction in both Cbl- and folate-deficient marrows.

Methylmalonic acid excretion (MMA)

An increase in the urinary excretion of MMA after an oral dose of 10 g valine is specific for Cbl deficiency. Under these circumstances normal subjects excrete a mean of 2 mg in the urine in the next 24 hours with a range of 1–15 mg. Specific assay involves ether extraction of the urine and assay of MMA by gas chromatography. There are a host of easier colorimetric methods described. These are satisfactory when there are large amounts of MMA in the urine but when the concentration is relatively low, false positive results due to other weak organic acids in urine occur. These methods are not recommended. A method using deuterium-labelled MMA and analysis by mass spectrometry [38] has made it possible to assay MMA in sera, even samples stored for some time, so that retrospective diagnosis is possible. It is rather complex for routine practice.

An increase in urinary MMA occurs in the majority of patients with Cbl deficiency, but the least anaemic with the highest Cbl levels do not have an increased excretion [39].

Following an injection of Cbl in a deficient patient there is a rapid decline in the amount of MMA excreted in the next 48 hours followed by a more gradual fall to normal excretion over the next 3–5 days. Folate therapy given to a Cbl-deficient patient had no effect on MMA excretion.

The test is particularly useful in children with megaloblastic anaemia where complex situations involving both MMA metabolism and methionine synthetase can occur singly or together (Chapter 14).

The stomach and gastric secretion

In the collection of gastric juice, the fasting gastric contents should be discarded and thereafter gastric secretion collected for 30 min, a gastric stimulant such as pentagastrin given and a further 30-min collection made. The volume and pH are measured and then pH brought to 10 with 40N–KOH to destroy pepsin, pH restored to about 7 with HCl and the juice stored at −20°C until assayed for IF content. Assay of IF is relatively easy to perform. Cobinamide added to an aliquot of gastric juice will block all R-binders so that when $[^{57}Co]B_{12}$ is added it will bind only to IF. Under these circumstances the binding of $[^{57}Co]B_{12}$ to gastric juice is a measure of its IF content. One unit of IF is contained in the volume of gastric juice binding 1 ng of $[^{57}Co]B_{12}$.

In pernicious anaemia the volume of unstimulated gastric secretion is low — 15–20 ml/hour as compared to 50–150 ml/hour in controls and there is no increase in output after a stimulant to secretion. HCl is absent in pernicious anaemia, the pH is usually 6–8 after a stimulant but occasionally can fall to about 4.0 in some patients who still have small numbers of residual parietal cells. Acid in the gastric juice excludes a diagnosis of pernicious anaemia.

The normal concentration of IF in the post-stimulant gastric juice sample is 14–114 units/ml. In pernicious anaemia IF is usually absent or may be present in a concentration of up to 6 units/ml. In terms of total output of IF among 75 patients with pernicious anaemia, 51 had none and 24 has less than 200 IF units/hour. Normal subjects excrete in excess of 1400 IF units/hour. However, patients with atrophic gastritis secrete intermediate amounts right down to the pernicious anaemia range in severe gastric atrophy (Fig. 4.2).

Endoscopy should be part of the normal investigation in pernicious anaemia to exclude gastric carcinoma, gastric carcinoid and polyps which are relatively frequent. It is usual to take a biopsy at the same time. Severe atrophic gastritis of the body of the stomach is the rule but in one-third of biopsies a few residual parietal cells are present. Significant numbers of parietal cells make a diagnosis of pernicious anaemia unlikely. The gastric antrum is normal except in pernicious ana-

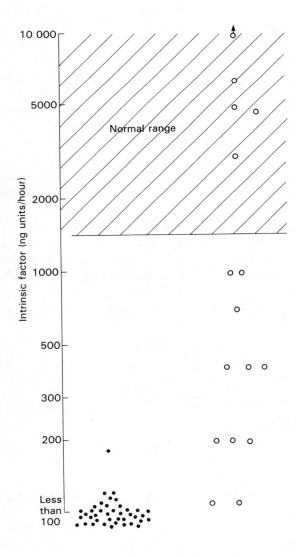

Fig. 4.2 The normal output of IF after pentagastrin stimulation is in excess of 1400 to over 10 000 units per hour (hatched area). Most patients with pernicious anaemia (●) do not have detectable amounts of IF but a few excrete up to 200 units in the hour. Patients with atrophic gastritis without pernicious anaemia (○) may secrete as little as do pernicious anaemia patients, but generally secrete more and patients with less severe gastritis secrete normal quantities.

emia accompanying hypogammaglobulinaemia when both body and antrum are atrophic.

Cobalamin absorption tests

The absorption of Cbl is a valuable and physiological test providing important clinical data when properly performed. It is usual to use $[^{57}Co]Cbl$ because this isotope gives the least amount of radiation to the patient and in terms of permissable dose over 200 tests could be performed in a single patient without reaching this level. Its counting characteristics are such that high counting rates are achieved with the standard test and is particularly useful for counting plasma radioactivity. There are several ways in which Cbl absorption can be tested.

Urinary excretion test (Schilling test)

The test is performed by giving 1 µg of Cbl containing about 0.5 µCi of $[^{57}Co]B_{12}$ by mouth and at the same time (some prefer to wait 1–2 hours) 1000 µg of non-radioactive cyanocobalamin (CNCbl) by injection. Some 85% of the CNCbl will be excreted into the urine. As only about 2 µg of the 1000 µg CNCbl will be attached to R-binder and TCII, the remainder will be unbound or free and this is filtered by the glomerulus and not reabsorbed by the renal tubules. The clearance of free Cbl is, in fact, an excellent measure of glomerular filtration rate. One-third of the $[^{57}Co]B_{12}$ reaching plasma from the gut will join the large pool of free Cbl and pass into the urine in the next 24 hours. Counting the $[^{57}Co]B_{12}$ in the 24-hour urine gives a reliable assessment of Cbl absorption. Normal subjects excrete more than 10% of the oral dose into urine in 24 hours (11–39%, mean 22%). Patients with pernicious anaemia excrete less than 10% and generally less than 7% (Table 4.2).

Table 4.2 Results of Cbl absorption tests using $[^{57}Co]B_{12}$, a urinary excretion method and a 1.0 µg dose of Cbl. Results are expressed as % excretion in urine of the oral dose. The flushing dose was 1000 µg CNCbl.

Controls	Pernicious anaemia	
	Dose alone	Dose + IF
11–39 (mean 22)	0–6.8	3.1–30.0 (mean 10.0)

Warning

The test is only valid if the urine collection is complete. Among hospital in-patients lost urine occurs in at least 25% of all tests. Collection is virtually never complete among the elderly. In infants a metabolic cot can be used to ensure complete collection, although some $[^{57}Co]B_{12}$ may pass into urine from faeces as this is passed at the same time.

The administration of other isotopes such as technecium may give falsely high counts. As these have a very short half-life recount of the urine after a few days may resolve the problem. Rarely the $[^{57}Co]B_{12}$ may be contaminated by ^{57}Co in other forms. These will pass into urine and give falsely high results.

Cyanocobalamin is used because the other form of Cbl available for parenteral injection, hydroxocobalamin (OHCbl), binds strongly to albumin and less of the dose is excreted into urine (average 29% of a 1000 μg dose). It may be that OHCbl is as satisfactory as CNCbl in Cbl absorption tests but this has not been demonstrated satisfactorily and, until it is, CNCbl should be used.

Other than in dietary Cbl lack in vegetarians, Cbl deficiency always arises from impaired Cbl absorption. Normal absorption therefore excludes Cbl deficiency. Other possible exceptions are the rare inherited abnormalities of Cbl metabolism.

Plasma radioactivity

The physiological absorption of Cbl leads to a peak plasma level between 8 and 12 hours after an oral dose. Thus if an oral dose in a Schilling test is given at 8 or 9 hours a blood sample collected at 17 hours should show peak radioactivity. Because of the high frequency of incomplete urine collections, the urinary excretion test for Cbl absorption must always be combined with measurement of plasma radioactivity. The plasma from 20 ml blood collected into any anticoagulant is satisfactory and is counted in an appropriate gamma counter.

With a 1.0 μg oral dose of $[^{57}Co]B_{12}$, the plasma radioactivity when a 1000 μg Cbl injection is given, ranges from 0.67 to 2.19% of the oral dose/litre plasma (mean 1.28). In pernicious anaemia the range is 0.02–0.42%. The test is very reliable and normal plasma radioactivity in the presence of a low urine excretion must be interpreted as normal Cbl absorption with incomplete urine collection.

The test is valid in patients with renal failure and is particularly useful in the elderly and perhaps incontinent patients.

Whole body counting

Where facilities are available this is a useful method of assessing Cbl absorption. $[^{58}Co]B_{12}$ is easier to count than $[^{57}Co]B_{12}$ but both can be used. A background count is made with the patient in the whole body counter, a dose of labelled Cbl is given and the patient recounted 30 min later. Finally retained

Cbl is assessed by a count made after 5 days or more. Normal subjects retain more than 30% of a 1 µg dose. The method is useful in out-patient practice. In hospital practice the urinary excretion and plasma radioactivity is preferred as the result is available sooner. Although whole body counting should be foolproof provided *bona fide* labelled Cbl is given, errors do occur probably due to careless setting of counting channels or not allowing a Cbl capsule to dissolve and pass down the gut.

Faecal excretion method   All faeces are collected for unabsorbed labelled Cbl after an oral dose. This primitive method is no longer used as few patients are willing or able to collect all stool samples into cans for 5 or more days. Results are the same as the whole body counts on the rare occasions when the stool collections are complete.

Comments   Cobalamin absorption tests can be repeated by giving the oral dose of Cbl with a source of IF. In patients with IF deficiency (pernicious anaemia, post-gastrectomy, simple atrophic gastritis) the results will be improved significantly. Patients with pernicious anaemia may show a relatively poor response to added IF because they may have IF antibodies in the GI tract or because long-standing Cbl deficiency in itself depresses Cbl absorption. The last problem should be corrected after a few months of Cbl therapy and a repeat Cbl absorption test with added IF should produce a much better Cbl absorption than initially. Steroids, even short-term, improve Cbl absorption in pernicious anaemia both by allowing some IF to be produced and by depressing immune factors.

When there is no improvement in Cbl absorption with a dose of IF, an intestinal lesion appears likely. This can be an abnormal bacterial flora in the gut or disease of the gut wall. In the former case a week's antibiotic (tetracycline or other wide spectrum antibiotic) will restore Cbl absorption at least temporarily.

Cbl labelled with two isotopes, $[^{57}Co]B_{12}$ and $[^{58}Co]B_{12}$, can be used together, the one being free and the second bound to IF. Because of the wide differences in the gamma emission the concentration of each isotope can be determined in a mixture. Since a normal subject has IF in the gastric juice, this will bind to the free Cbl. Thus both forms of cobalamin will be absorbed to an equal extent and the ratio of the two isotopes in either urine or plasma is unity. However, if the subject lacks IF the free Cbl will not be absorbed to a significant degree and the ratio will change. Only a sample of urine rather than a complete collection is required. The results of the test are often obscured because of an exchange of Cbl on IF so that the free Cbl acquires some IF. Thus equivocal results may occur [40].

Another variant of the use of Cbl labelled with two isotopes is in the investigation of pancreatic disease. One isotope is bound to IF and the other to R-binder [41]. At an acid pH much of the dietary Cbl in the stomach binds to R-binder and, proteolytic enzymes from the pancreas, by digesting R-binder, release Cbl to bind to IF. This does not occur in pancreatic disease so that malabsorption of Cbl bound to R-binder occurs. Thus normally if two isotopes are given, $[^{57}Co]Cbl-IF$ and $[^{58}Co]Cbl-R$-binder using the urinary excretion test, results are 21.2% and 16.2%, respectively. In intestinal malabsorption the absorption of both is depressed equally. In symptomatic pancreatic disease the urinary excretion of Cbl–IF is 16.3% but of Cbl-R binder only 1.0%. It should be emphasized that impaired Cbl absorption in pancreatic disease is never of sufficient severity to cause Cbl deficiency.

Another somewhat ill-conceived variant of the Cbl absorption test involves administration to the patient of Cbl bound to chick serum. This is an avid Cbl binder — so much so that the Cbl is virtually unavailable to normal subjects. Thus in the urinary excretion test normal subjects excrete about 20% of a 1 µg dose of Cbl. When the Cbl is bound to chick serum this falls to less than 1–6% of the dose [42,43]. Results of less than 1% are abnormal. Abnormal results are obtained in patients with achlorhydria, that is patients with simple atrophic gastritis and pernicious anaemia. The absorption is not improved by adding IF to the $[^{57}Co]B_{12}$–chick serum complex but is improved by giving HCl and/or pepsin [44]. Since patients with simple atrophic gastritis often have a low Cbl level but still normal Cbl absorption, an abnormal result in the Cbl-chick serum absorption test has been interpreted as being a more sensitive test for IF deficiency. This is not correct. If the absorption of Cbl is normal, the patient is able to secrete more than the 500 IF units necessary to achieve this absorption and this is the reason why they are and remain haematologically normal. The low Cbl–chick serum absorption reflects achlorhydria and absent pepsinogen activation. It is of doubtful clinical value.

The causes of impaired Cbl absorption are shown in Table 4.3.

Table 4.3 Causes of cobalamin malabsorption

Congenital causes
Abnormal or absent intrinsic factor
Vitamin B_{12} malabsorption (Imerslund-Gräsbeck)
Transcobalamin II deficiency

Acquired causes
Gastric lesion
Atrophy (pernicious anaemia and simple atrophic gastritis)
Subtotal or total gastrectomy
Caustic cicatrization
Gastric bypass

Intestinal causes
Luminal
Abnormal gut flora associated with:
Blind loops
Strictures
Entero–entero anastomosis
Fistulae between gut segments
Small intestinal diverticulae
Poorly functioning gastroenterostomy
Reduced gut motility (scleroderma, Whipple's Disease, post-vagotomy, ganglion-blocking drugs)
Gut resections
Regional ileitis
Abnormal pH (Zollinger-Ellison)
Pancreatic insufficiency (chronic pancreatisis, cystic fibrosis)
Giardiasis, *D. latum*
Intrinsic-factor antibody forming Ig-IF complex.

Disease of gut wall
Gluten sensitivity
Tropical sprue
Regional ileitis
Infiltration (mastocytosis)
Ileal bypass or resection
Following deficiency of B_{12} or folate
Radiation damage
Drugs, including alcohol

Intrinsic-factor antibodies

The presence of antibodies to gastric IF is a useful adjunct to the diagnosis of pernicious anaemia. They are detected because, by binding to the site on IF normally occupied by Cbl, they reduce the binding of $[^{57}Co]B_{12}$ in an aliquot of gastric juice (Fig. 4.3). Other antibodies react with sites on the IF molecule other than the Cbl binding site. They are less common and more difficult to detect.

IF antibodies are present in about 57% of sera from pernicious anaemia patients. Antibodies are also present in gastric secretion and cell-mediated immunity against IF is demonstrable in about 80% of patients [45]. In practice only antibodies to IF are useful. The presence of such antibodies is not entirely unique to pernicious anaemia. They can occur rarely in the absence of pernicious anaemia as in thyroid disease, simple

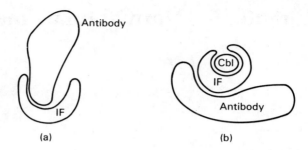

Fig. 4.3 Humoral antibodies to IF are present in over half the patients with pernicious anaemia. The common type prevents Cbl binding to IF and is presumed to react with the Cbl-binding site on the molecule (a). Less commonly an antibody that reacts with the IF–Cbl complex (b) is present.

atrophic gastritis and in relatives of patients with pernicious anaemia. Seven-year follow-up of such patients did not show any transition into pernicious anaemia [46]. Furthermore, nearly half the patients with pernicious anaemia lack the antibody. Nevertheless IF antibodies make it very likely that the patient has pernicious anaemia. Almost all such patients also have parietal-cell antibodies.

Response to cobalamin therapy

A haematological and clinical response to Cbl therapy alone is good evidence that the patient had Cbl deficiency. The evidence is more impressive if the dose of Cbl is 2 µg day by injection. In dietary Cbl deficiency proof of the diagnosis is response to say 5 µg Cbl daily given by mouth. Ideally, with large doses of Cbl a reticulocyte peak should be reached on day 5, 6 or 7 after starting therapy and the red cell count should exceed 3 million in the third week (Fig. 7.1). With small doses of Cbl, parenterally or orally, reticulocyte responses are more muted but haematological normality should be restored. Despite some claims in the literature to the contrary, patients with folate deficiency do not respond in any significant way to Cbl therapy.

Chapter 5   Normal folate metabolism

Folates, present in all living cells, are essential for cell replication by virtue of their role in the synthesis of nucleic acid bases.

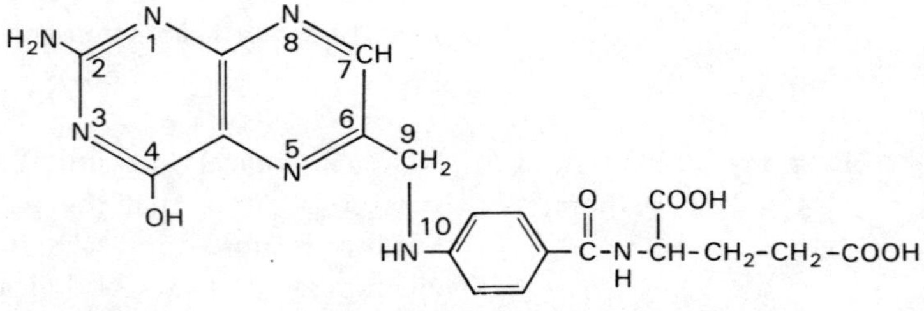

Fig. 5.1 Pteroylglutamic acid (PteGlu).

Pteridine   para-aminobenzoic acid   Glutamic acid

Biochemistry   Pteroylglutamic acid (Fig. 5.1) consists of a double-ringed pteridine portion, joined to para-aminobenzoic acid (PABA) and to glutamic acid. This is the stable pharmacological analogue. The physiological analogues are derivatives of tetra-hydropteroylglutamic acid. The shorthand for pteroylglutamic acid is PteGlu; the tetrahydro-analogue is designated H_4PteGlu. The four hydrogens are on carbons 5, 6, 7 and 8 so that designation is 5,6,7,8–H_4PteGlu.

Once folate enters the cell, additional glutamic acid residues are added — these compounds are called pteroylpolygluta-mates or folate polyglutamates designated as H_4PteGlu$_n$. If the number of glutamic acid residues is known as in tetrahy-dropteroylpentaglutamate, it is designated H_4PteGlu$_5$ (Fig. 5.2).

In addition to being reduced (Fig. 5.3) and polyglutamated, folates may carry a transferable single carbon unit, either formyl (–CHO), methenyl (=CH–), methylene (–CH$_2$–) or methyl (–CH$_3$). Formyl is carried on nitrogen 10 so that the compound is designated 10–CHO–H_4PteGlu, and methyl on nitrogen 5 the compound being 5–CH$_3$–H_4PteGlu. The re-

46

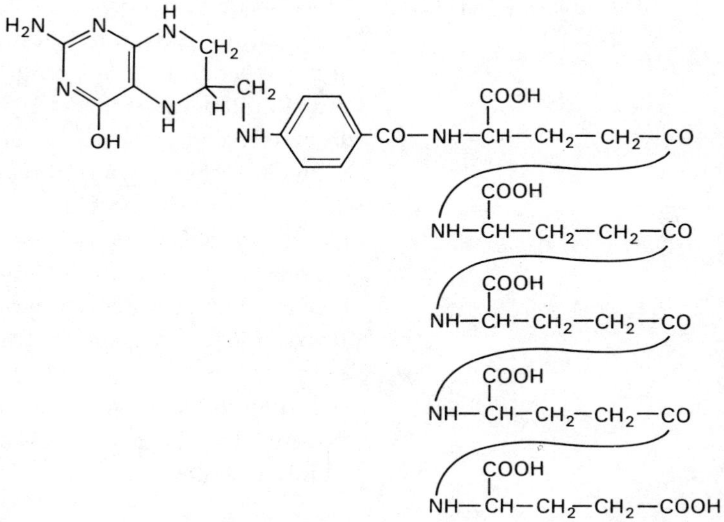

Fig. 5.2 Tetrahydropteroylpentaglutamate (H₄PteGlu₅).

maining two compounds are carried as bridge compounds
attached both to nitrogens 5 and 10 as 5,10–CH=H₄PteGlu or
5,10–CH₂–H₄PteGlu. Histidine catabolism yields a further
1–C unit as a formimino–(–CH=NH) which contributes a
methenyl group.

An additional folate analogue arises druing the course of
thymidine synthesis, namely dihydropteroylglutamic acid
designated as H₂PteGlu.

The oxidized analogue, pteroylglutamic acid is a stable
compound. The reduced compounds are unstable and readily
oxidized even by atmospheric oxygen and this may be accompanied by cleavage of the molecule at the 9–10 bond.
Natural folates are protected by reducing agents such as ascorbate. Mammals are unable to synthesize folates and hence
these have to be obtained from the diet. However, the parent
compound is modified within the animal cell by a variety of
enzymes.

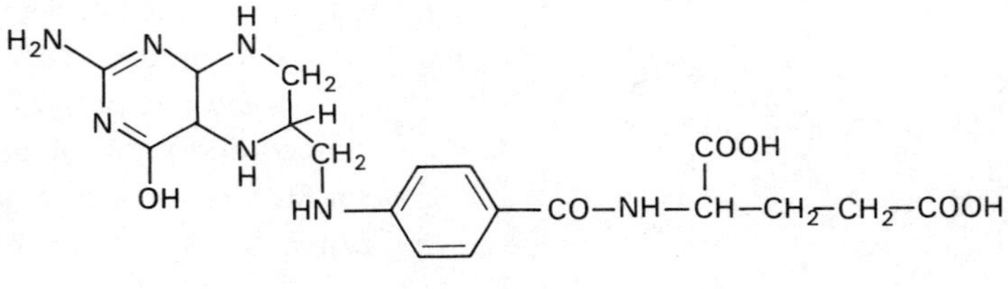

Fig. 5.3 Tetrahydropteroyl-
glutamic acid or tetrahydrofolic
acid (H₄PteGlu).

Dihydrofolate reductase This enzyme converts $H_2PteGlu$ into $H_4PteGlu$. Dihydrofolate arises during the methylation of deoxyuridine to thymidine. In this reaction a $-CH_2-$ group is transferred to deoxyuridine and simultaneously the $-CH_2-$ is reduced to methyl the hydrogens being donated by $H_4PteGlu$ which then becomes $H_2PteGlu$. The enzyme dihydrofolate reductase regenerates $H_4PteGlu$ using NADPH as the hydrogen donor (Fig. 5.4). The enzyme from a variety of species has been characterized in great detail. It is the site of binding of folate antagonists such as methotrexate and pyrimethamine and, with bacterial dihydrofolate reductase, of trimethoprim. The same enzyme is probably concerned with reduction of pharmacological folic acid (pteroylglutamic acid) to $H_4PteGlu$ as it is capable of reducing PteGlu at a slow rate to $H_2PteGlu$ and $H_2PteGlu$ rapidly to $H_4PteGlu$.

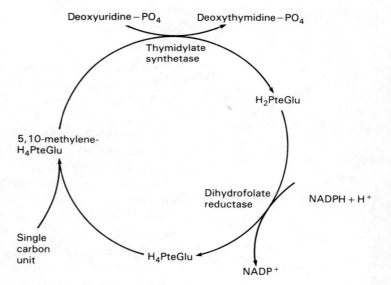

Fig. 5.4 Dihydropteroylglutamic acid ($H_2PteGlu$) arises during the synthesis of thymidine when reduction of $-CH_2-$ from methylene H_4folate to the $-CH_3$ of thymidine requires hydrogens from $H_4PteGlu$. Dihydrofolate reductase regenerates $H_2PteGlu$ to $H_4PteGlu$.

Pteroylpolyglutamate The glutamic acid residues in folate polyglutamates are joined
conjugase (hydrolase) in peptide ($-CO-NH-$) bonds but unlike the alpha linkage of amino acids in proteins the gamma carboxyl of glutamic acid is utilized. Enzymes that remove glutamic acid residues are present in most tissues. They are unusual in so far as they function optimally at pH 4.5, like other lysosomal enzymes and are concerned with folate polyglutamate catabolism.

A second hydrolase acting at about pH 7 has been identified in the brush border of the enterocyte [47]. This enzyme is probably concerned with the physiological absorption of folate polyglutamates. These must be converted into monoglutamate by the removal of all glutamic acid residues in excess of one in the enterocyte or the gut lumen. The enzyme is present in high concentration in human intestinal mucosa.

Pteroylpolyglutamate synthetase

This enzyme is present in most cells and is concerned with adding glutamic acid residues to folate. The resulting polyglutamate is the active coenzyme and is retained in the cell unlike pteroylmonoglutamates which can be excreted into bile and be recirculated [48]. Methotrexate can serve as a substrate for this enzyme which converts it into methotrexatepolyglutamate. The preferred substrate is either H_4PteGlu or CHO–H_4PteGlu but normally not CH_3–H_4PteGlu. Cell lines which lack pteroylpolyglutamate synthetase can only grow if performed glycine, adenosine and thymidine are supplied indicating that a polyglutamate coenzyme is the functional form.

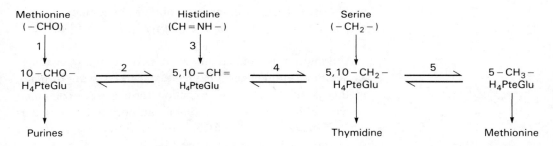

Fig 5.5 Folate transfers single carbon units and the state of reduction of these carbon units is altered by a series of multifunctional enzymes. It is probable that methionine is the main source of formate (–CHO) required for purine synthesis. Formyltetrahydrofolate synthetase transfers formate to tetrahydrofolate (1). Formate is reduced to methenyl by 5,10-methenyl tetrahydrofolate cyclohydrolase (2). Methenyl can also arise from histidine as a formimino (CH=NH–) group (3). The enzymes are 5-formiminotetrahydrofolate dehydrogenase and 5-formiminotetrahydrofolate cyclohydrolase (3). The methenyl group is further reduced to methylene by 5, 10-methylenetetrahydrofolate dehydrogenase (4) and this is the stage of reduction required for thymidine synthesis. Finally, methylene is reduced to methyl by 5,10-methylenetetrahydrofolate reductase (5). The methyl group is required for methionine synthesis.

Enzymes concerned with oxidation/reduction of single-carbon units

The role of the folate coenzymes is in transfer of single-carbon (1–C) units. In purine synthesis the 1–C unit is required as formate, for thymidine synthesis it is required as methylene and for methionine synthesis as methyl. Interconverting enzymes change the state of reduction of these 1–carbon units (Fig. 5.5).

Formyltetrahydrofolate synthetase transfers active formate to $H_4PteGlu$. The formate can then be oxidized to CO_2 *(10–formyltetrahydrofolate dehydrogenase)* if not required, it can be used in purine synthesis, or it can be reduced to methenyl (–CH=) by the enzyme *5,10–methenyltetrahydrofolate cyclohydrolase*. This folate analogue has no synthetic role and is a step to the synthesis of 5,10–methylenetetrahydrofolate, the enzyme being *5,10–methylenetetrahydrofolate dehydrogenase*. A CH_2–group more commonly arises by the transfer of a 1–C unit from serine to $H_4PteGlu$. The –CH_2– may then be transferred to deoxyuridine in thymidine synthesis or it may be reduced to methyl by *5,10–methylenetetrahydrofolate reductase*. The methyl group is normally transferred to homocysteine to form methionine. All but the last of these enzymes function in both directions, that is they will both oxidize or reduce the relevant 1–C unit. The exception *in vitro* is methylene reductase where the reaction strongly favours methylfolate synthesis. *In vivo,* however, elevation of the methionine level causes rapid oxidation of the methyl group to formyl and CO_2.

Although it is convenient to regard all these enzymes as separate entities the enzymes concerned with formate, methenyl and methylene formation form a large combined enzyme although each component can be influenced separately. Thus inactivation of Cbl is followed by a rise in formyl synthetase activity, a fall in cyclohydrolase activity but no change in dehydrogenase activity.

Function of folate coenzymes

Folates function in the transfer of 1–C units in the synthesis of purines, thymidine and methionine. The source of these 1–C units is serine, methionine, formate and histidine.

Serine transhydroxymethylase

This enzyme catalyses the transfer of the β-carbon of serine to $H_4PteGlu$. It is the general view that this is the major source of 1–C units (Fig. 5.6). Glycine too can donate its alpha carbon unit to the folate pool.

5–formiminotetrahydrofolate transferase/cyclodeaminase

This is another multifunctional enzyme. 5–CHNH–$H_4PteGlu$ (5–formiminoH$_4$PteGlu) arises in the course of histidine catabolism, the 1–C in the –CH=NH group arising from carbon–2 of the imidazole ring of histidine. Histidine catabolism (Fig. 5.7) leads to the formation of formiminoglutamic acid. Its

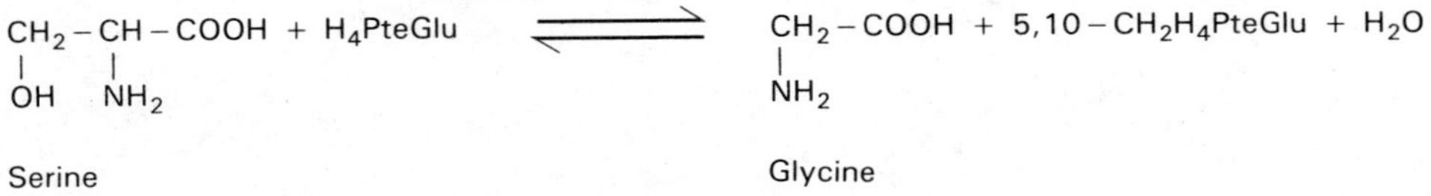

$$CH_2-CH-COOH + H_4PteGlu \rightleftharpoons CH_2-COOH + 5,10-CH_2H_4PteGlu + H_2O$$

(Serine: CH_2 bears OH, CH bears NH_2) (Glycine: CH_2 bears NH_2)

Serine   Glycine

Fig. 5.6 Transhydroxymethylase *in vitro* converts serine to glycine with release of a single carbon at the methylene state of reduction. It is difficult to demonstrate this reaction *in vivo*.

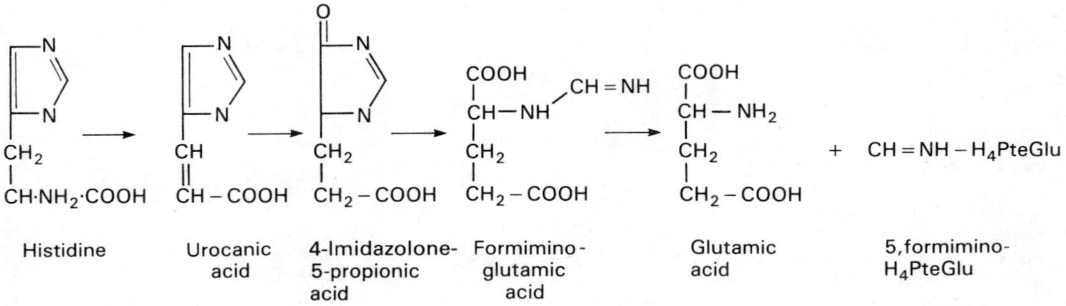

Histidine → Urocanic acid → 4-Imidazolone-5-propionic acid → Formimino-glutamic acid → Glutamic acid + $CH=NH-H_4PteGlu$ (5,formimino-$H_4PteGlu$)

Fig. 5.7 The catabolism of histidine to glutamic acid via formiminoglutamic acid and release of a 1-carbon unit. It is not an important source of 1-carbon units.

further metabolism involves transfer of the formimino group to $H_4PteGlu$ by the transferase and removal of the $=NH$ group by the cyclodeaminase. The resulting folate compound is $5,10-CH=H_4PteGlu$. The excretion of formiminoglutamic acid in urine particularly after an oral histidine load, has been used as a test for folate deficiency.

Methionine as a source of 1–C unit

Methionine is largely converted into S–adenosylmethionine. One of the pathways that S–adenosylmethionine can follow is in polyamine metabolism (Fig. 5.8) when it supplies a 3–carbon chain for the formation of spermidine and putrescine. The 5′–methylthioadenosine portion remaining is regenerated into methionine and 1 mol of formate is released for each mole of methionine produced (Fig. 5.9). This has been shown to serve as a source of formate, e.g. for purine synthesis. In addition the methyl group of methionine can be oxidized to formate and CO_2. This step too must pass through folate.

Purine synthesis

Carbons 2 and 8 of the purine ring are contributed by 10–formyl$H_4PteGlu$. An early step is addition of 1–C to glycinamide ribonucleotide which becomes C–8 of the purine

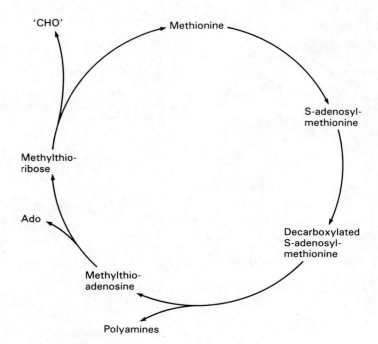

Fig. 5.8 The pathway by which methionine donates a formate unit via methylthioribose. Between 0.5 and 1.0 mmol of methionine per day enters the polyamine pathway. This is probably enough to meet mans' formate requirements.

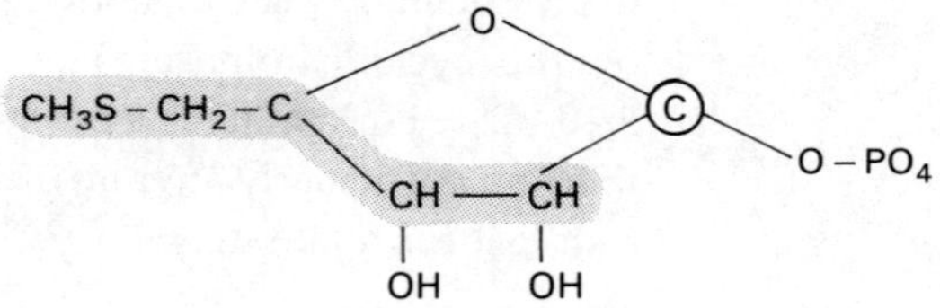

Fig. 5.9 Methylthioribose is regenerated into methionine the CH_3–S moiety being derived from the original methionine molecule. The rest of the methionine comes from ribose. For each mole of methionine formed a mole of active formate is released. Regenerated methionine is the elongated hatched area and formate the circle.

nucleus (Fig. 5.10). The enzyme is glycinamide ribonucleotide (GAR–) transformylase. The closure of the purine ring is brought about by the addition of a 1–C unit to 5–amino–4–imidazole carboxamide ribonucleotide (AICAR) to yield inosinic acid (Fig. 5.11). The enzyme is AICAR transformylase.

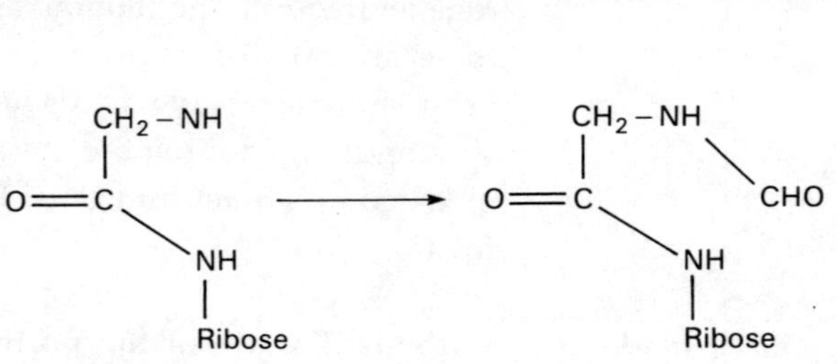

Fig. 5.10 Carbon-8 of the purine nucleus is donated as formate from 10-formylH₄folate.

Glycinamide ribonucleotide

Formylglycinamide ribonucleotide

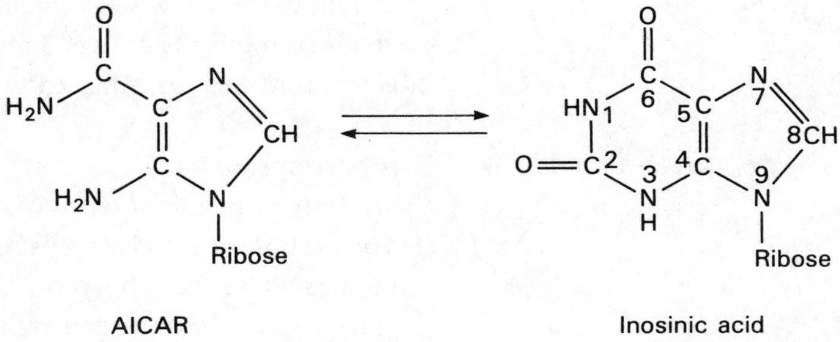

Fig. 5.11 The closure of the purine nucleus by formate supplying carbon-2 from 10-formylH$_4$PteGlu.

AICAR

Inosinic acid

Thymidine synthesis

The enzyme thymidylate synthetase transfers a 1–C unit from 5,10–CH$_2$–H$_4$PteGlu to deoxyuridine monophosphate. The reduction of the methylene group to methyl is achieved by transfer of hydrogens 5 and 6 of the pteridine ring so that folate becomes 7,8–H$_2$PteGlu (Fig. 5.12).

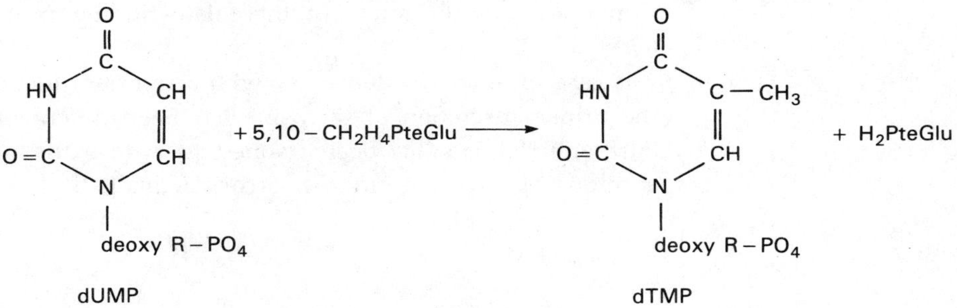

dUMP

dTMP

Fig. 5.12 The methylation of deoxyuridine-monophosphate to deoxythymidine-monophosphate.

Methionine synthesis

The *de novo* synthesis of methionine involves both Cbl and folate coenzymes directly. Other effects of Cbl deficiency on folate metabolism are largely secondary to an impairment of this crucial pathway. The enzyme is methionine synthetase or homocysteine methyltransferase. The reaction (Fig. 3.2) involves the transfer of a methyl group from methylH$_4$folate to Cbl to form methylCbl. MethylCbl is the coenzyme of methionine synthetase. Thereafter the methyl group is transferred to homocysteine. Cbl is required in the Cob[I]alamin or fully reduced state. Initially S–adenosylmethionine is required (at least *in vitro*) to prime the reaction but thereafter transfer of the methyl group proceeds without S–adenosylmethionine. In liver there is a second pathway that can methylate homocysteine namely, betaine homocysteine methyltransferase wherein betaine provides the methyl group instead of methylH$_4$folate. The betaine pathway, however, is absent from tissues other than liver.

Porphyrin synthesis

Uroporphyrinogen III is the precursor of haem. It is formed from four porphobilinogen (pyrrole) units. Two enzymes are involved but the precise steps remain unresolved. One of these enzymes in uroporphyrinogen III co-synthase. The enzyme has a co-factor which appears to be 5–CH$_3$–H$_4$PteGlu$_7$ and it was suggested that it participated in an intramolecular re-arrangement leading to formation of Uro III [49].

Methyl group oxidation in dimethylglycine and sarcosine

Dimethylglycine and sarcosine dehydrogenases in mitochondria both carry tightly bound folatepolyglutamate. Both mediate the oxidation of the methyl group to formaldehyde. The formaldehyde is taken up by tetrahydrofolate polyglutamates to yield 5,10–CH$_2$–H$_4$PteGlu$_5$ (Fig. 5.13). These enzymes account for much of the folate-binding protein of liver [50,51].

A case of folic acid deficiency with a transient increase in the urinary excretion of sarcosine has been described [52]. Further folic acid has been claimed to reduce the urinary excretion of sarcosine in hypersarcosinaemia [53].

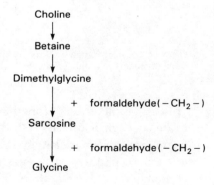

Fig. 5.13 The loss of methyl groups from choline to glycine. Both dimethylglycine and sarcosine can oxidize their methyl groups to yield 5,10-methyleneH$_4$folate.

Initiation of protein synthesis

The amino acid sequence on proteins starts with formyl-methionine on to which subsequent amino acids are attached. The formylation of methionyl-transfer RNA is through the donation of a 1–C by 10–formyl–H$_4$PteGlu [54].

Distribution, intake and requirement of folate

Folates are present in all foodstuffs of both plant and animal origin. The bulk of folates are methyl or formylpolyglutamates and all are H$_4$– or H$_2$PteGlu$_n$ analogues. Earlier tables setting out folate content of foodstuffs were grossly misleading because the assay procedures failed to recognize the labile nature of folate and the requirement that the assay procedure should respond equally to all the folate analogues in the diet. Recent tables are probably more reliable [55–57]. Folates are labile in so far as there is considerable loss during cooking of food as well as during the period of storage. Folates are lost on exposure to ultraviolet light. On the other hand folates are protected by reducing agents such as ascorbate. Under some circumstances 90% of the folate can be lost but more usually it is 40–50%. The data on dietary intake are compiled on cooked foods.

In Canada the mean daily folate intake is 205 μg/day for men and 149 μg/day for women [58] which is about 3 μg/kg body weight. In the United Kingdom the daily folate intake assessed over a 3-year period ranged from 210 to 213 μg [59]. With this mean folate intake about 8% of adults have red cell folate concentrations below the normal range. The folate distribution among different classes of foodstuffs during a single day is shown in Table 5.1. These data indicate that all components of a diet contribute some folate although some sources particularly liver are richer than others.

Table 5.1 Folate distribution (μg) in different classes of foodstuffs

Meat	13.9
Liver	26.6
Milk	34.0
Eggs, cheese, yoghurt	18.3
Vegetables	64.1
Fruit	24.6
Bread	19.5
Cereal, cake, sweets, beer	24.1

Cow's milk contains about 50 μg folate/l. Pasteurization does not reduce this but does destroy ascorbate. Reheating pasteurized milk, or milk powder that has been prepared with heat, reduces the folate to 10 μg/l. Powdered dried milk when reconstituted generally contains 30–40 μg/l, although there is much variation. Human breast milk too has about 50 μg folate/l.

In general, reduced folate monoglutamates are almost completely absorbed and these constitute about half the folate in a cooked meal. There is uncertainty about the availability of polyglutamates but current evidence is that 50–70% is absorbed.

An expert committee of the FAO/WHO recommended a daily folate intake of 3.1 µg/kg which is equivalent to 200 µg PteGlu for a 65 kg man and 170 µg for a 55 kg woman. The amount was considered to be a safe level of intake to cover the needs of 95% of the population.

Intestinal absorption of folate

The physiological processes for the intestinal absorption of folates convert the folate analogues present in a mixed diet to 5-methyltetrahydrofolate which is delivered to portal blood. Large doses of unphysiological folate analogues such as milligram amounts of pteroylglutamic acid (PteGlu) bypass these pathways and reach the blood unchanged.

There is good evidence that there is a specific receptor on the enterocyte for folates and that this may be lacking in congenital folate malabsorption, a disorder in which folate, even in very large doses, is not absorbed. A protein (MW +100 000) has been isolated from the brush border of rat gut [60] which binds short-chain folates rather than longer-chain ones. Absorption of folates involves the removal of glutamic acid residues in excess of one, reduction of the pteridine ring to the tetrahydro-form if required, formylation of H_4PteGlu and reduction of the formyl group to methyl and passage of $5-CH_3H_4$PteGlu to portal blood (Fig. 5.14). The hydrolase enzymes that cleave glutamic acid residues probably operate in the gut lumen or possibly the surface of the brush border [47]. The other changes all occur in the enterocyte [61,62]. When labelled H_2PteGlu is given *orally* to man labelled CH_3-H_4PteGlu only appears in blood. If, however, labelled H_2PteGlu is given by *injection* it disappears from the blood and exchanges with tissue unlabelled CH_3-H_4PteGlu which appears in blood. Methyltetrahydrofolate itself is absorbed unchanged.

Once absorbed most of the folate reaches the liver. Some may be excreted into bile and undergo an enterohepatic circulation. This would appear to be the mechanism for recirculating folate. Another portion of the folate is converted to either tetrahydrofolate or formyltetrahydrofolate following transfer of the methyl group to homocysteine. These two analogues are equally effective substrates for folate polyglutamate synthesis which is the next step in folate assimilation in the cell. Small amounts of folate appear in urine — less than 10 µg/day.

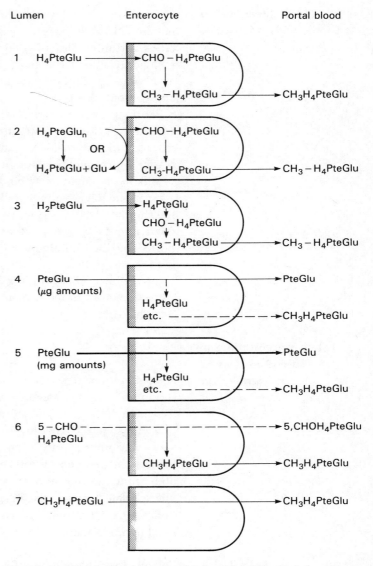

Fig. 5.14 In the intestinal absorption of dietary folate $H_4PteGlu$ is formylated and formate converted to methyl so that only 5-methyltetrahydrofolate enters portal blood (1). In the case of folatepolyglutamates, glutamic acid residues in excess of one are removed (2). Dihydrofolate is converted to tetrahydrofolate (3). Pteroylglutamic acid itself is not a physiological analogue. In small amount some is reduced and converted to 5-methylH_4folate but most is absorbed unchanged (4). With larger doses of pteroylglutamic acid most is absorbed unchanged (5). 5-formylH_4folate (folinic acid) is largely converted to methylH_4folate but a small proportion is absorbed unchanged (6). Methylfolate enters portal blood unchanged (7).

Internal transport of folate

The role of the enterohepatic circulation of folate has been mentioned. Cells have a membrane-associated protein that binds and internalizes 5-methyltetrahydrofolate [63]. Immunologically a similar folate-binding protein is present in milk and human placenta. Binders are also present in kidney cells and choroid plexus.

Serum has two folate binders. One is a high-affinity binder with a very low capacity that binds PteGlu in preference to physiological analogues and the second is a low-affinity binder which may be albumin.

Milk has a potent folate binder, the role of which may be to concentrate folate into the milk. The folate-binding protein in the choroid plexus specifically transports 5-methyltetrahydrofolate into the CSF [64]. Other folate analogues are not transported by the choroid plexus binder although PteGlu will bind to this protein.

Intracellular folate-binding proteins appear to be apoenzymes involved in folate metabolism and are present in both mitochondria and cytosol [65].

Folate concentrations in blood and tissues

Serum folate

Folate in plasma or serum is largely $5-CH_3H_4PteGlu$ but since serum does support some growth of *Str. faecalis* which cannot use methylfolate, it is likely that some formyl–$H_4PteGlu$ is present as well. Higher levels of formylfolates are present in sera from other species such as the rat. The level of serum folate is maintained by intake of methylfolate from the gut both from the diet and by an enterohepatic circulation of methylfolate through the biliary tract. The normal range is difficult to define with precision but is generally given as 3–20 ng/ml in man.

Red cell folate

Folate in red blood cells (RBCs) is almost entirely $5,CH_3–H_4PteGlu$. About 60–70% is in the form of folate polyglutamate with pentaglutamate predominating. The remaining one-third is directly available for microbiological assay suggesting that it is a monoglutamate. The concentration of folate in red cells ranges from 140 to 450 ng/ml packed red cells. Folate is incorporated into the developing erythroblast in the marrow. Reticulocytes have a significantly higher folate content than older red cells and presumably must lose some folate during maturation. The residual folate in RBCs has no metabolic role and remains unchanged in the RBCs until their demise 110 days later.

Cerebrospinal fluid folate

CSF folate concentrations are several times higher than in plasma indicating an important role for folate in the CNS. Not only is the CSF folate level higher than serum but there is considerable passage of methylfolate through the CSF and one-fifth of an intravenous 300 µg dose of labelled methylfolate given to man appeared in the CSF 4 hours later [66]. The folate level in CSF ranges from about 15 to 60 ng/ml.

Liver folate

There is a wide range of liver folate concentrations in samples obtained either at surgery or via percutaneous biopsy ranging from 0.7 to 17 µg/g. However, subjects with normal values for other parameters of folate status have liver folate concentrations greater than 4.4 µg/g. The mean folate value for liver is 7.1 µg/g of wet liver.

Chapter 6   Assessment of folate status

Diagnosis of folate deficiency depends on the following.
   Measurement of serum folate.
   Measurement of red cell folate.
   Measurement of tissue folate.
   Urinary formiminoglutamic acid excretion.
   Deoxyuridine suppression test.
   Response to folate.
   Exclusion of Cbl deficiency.
   Tests for folate absorption.
Some of these methods are appropriate for assessing sub-clinical deficiency states in haematologically normal subjects. Others are applicable to patients with megaloblastic haemopoiesis.

Serum folate

A low serum folate is to be found in almost all patients with folate deficiency. However, a low serum folate is also commonly encountered in ill patients who do not have any problems with haemopoiesis. Indeed, this may be the case in about one-third of such patients. It is probable that such patients are in negative folate balance, that is, there is reduced entry of folate from dietary sources. It would require many months of a reduced folate intake to produce significant deficiency [67]. Because of the very high frequency of low serum folate values in ill patients, this test is of limited diagnostic value. It should be added that a normal or raised serum folate occurs in 90% of patients with untreated pernicious anaemia. Normal serum folate in megaloblastic anaemia, not due to a haemolysed serum sample, is a pointer against folate deficiency. High serum folates may be found in patients with an abnormal intestinal gut flora.

Red cell folate

On the other hand a low red cell folate level is unequivocal evidence of folate deficiency. A low red cell folate is the consequence of several months of reduced folate supply. In some situations, as in megaloblastic anaemia in pregnancy, sufficient time may not have elapsed for the red cell folate to have fallen into a low range before megaloblastosis has supervened. Thus the red cell folate, while declining, may still be in the low normal range. Radioassay methods consistently record higher red cell folate levels within the normal range than *L.casei* assay but both show better agreement at low red cell folate values.

A raised reticulocyte count may give a too optimistic assessment of folate status. Thus in megaloblastic anaemia accompanying a haemolytic anaemia, liver folate levels may be extremely low but, because of the higher folate content of reticulocytes, the red cell folate may still be normal [7]. Transfusion of normal blood can produce a misleading pattern as well since, by virtue of the folate content of the transfused cells, normal red cell folate values can be restored although tissue deficiency persists. Serum folate is not affected by transfusion. In Herbert's study in which a very low dietary folate intake was maintained, serum folate fell within a few weeks whereas red cell folate only declined after 18 weeks [67].

Liver folate

On occasion a sample of liver, either as a percutaneous biopsy or biopsy taken during laparotomy, is available. In megaloblastic anaemia due to folate deficiency the folate level is 1 μg/g of wet liver or less. The normal mean value is 7.1 μg/g.

Urinary formiminoglutamic acid (Figlu) excretion

The metabolism of histidine yields a 1-carbon unit as a formimino (–CH=NH) group which is taken up by $H_4PteGlu$. In folate deficiency this pathway is impaired leading to an increased urinary excretion of Figlu especially if the pathway has been stressed by an oral histidine dose (15 g of L–histidine). Under these circumstances the urinary excretion exceeds 17 mg in 8 hours and is often very much more than this. As a test for folate deficiency it has lost popularity because it is also abnormal in Cbl deficiency and in many ill patients without primary folate problems as in thyrotoxicosis and congestive cardiac failure. Further, not uncommonly, the pathway of histidine catabolism does not progress beyond the first step which is cleavage of the imidazole ring of histidine to urocanic acid (Fig. 5.7). Thus urocanic acid rather than Figlu appears in urine. The test is of little value in pregnancy because of an altered renal threshold for histidine and a slower transport of oral histidine into portal blood and of equally little value in patients taking anticonvulsant drugs because enzyme induction changes the rates of catabolism [7]. When there is an increased excretion it is normalized within about 5 days of folate therapy.

Deoxyuridine suppression test

This test is always abnormal when there is megaloblastic haemopoiesis due to either Cbl or folate deficiency. Failure to produce any correction at all by adding Cbl, but correction with folinic acid, indicates folate deficiency as the cause.

Haematological response to folate

Unlike treatment with Cbl, all patients with megaloblastic anaemia respond to folate given in the relatively large doses which it is customary to use in clinical practice, namely 5–15 mg daily. However, when the dose of folate is reduced to about 200 µg daily, a haematological response occurs only in folate-deficient patients. Reticulocyte responses are suboptimal on this small dose but there should be a significant increase in haemoglobin and RBC count over several weeks. Long-term folate in Cbl deficiency is undesirable since it can aggravate a neuropathy. But in the short term, that is, over a few weeks, on such untoward effect occurs.

Exclusion of cobalamin deficiency

In populations where both Cbl deficiency or folate deficiency can produce megaloblastic anaemia, the exclusion of Cbl deficiency by demonstrating a normal serum Cbl level and/or normal Cbl absorption, is good evidence that the deficiency is due to folate. On occasion megaloblastic anaemia develops in a patient already receiving Cbl injections when the cause must be folate deficiency.

Folate absorption tests

The only situation where a test for folate absorption is essential is in the diagnosis of congenital folate malabsorption. This disorder presents as a severe megaloblastic anaemia in the first 3 months of life. These children are totally unable to absorb any folate analogue and have impaired transport of folate into the CSF. Thus normally an oral dose of 5 mg PteGlu to a 3-month-old child will be followed 1 hour later by a high plasma folate exceeding 100 ng/ml. In children with congenital folate malabsorption there is barely a detectable rise in plasma folate.

Folate absorption tests are not required in normal clinical practice since other simple tests of intestinal function are available. Its role lies in research situations and the methods are set out elsewhere [7].

Chapter 7   The response to therapy in megaloblastic anaemia

Assessment of the response to specific therapy in megaloblastic anaemia is important for several reasons. Firstly, it provides evidence that diagnosis of the deficiency is correct. Secondly, an inadequate response indicates that either diagnosis is wrong or that complicating factors have been overlooked. Thirdly, an understanding of the events in the response throws light on the pathophysiology of the underlying disease process.

Optimal haematological response

Because there is an accumulation of early megaloblasts in the marrow, the provision of a maximal dose of either Cbl or

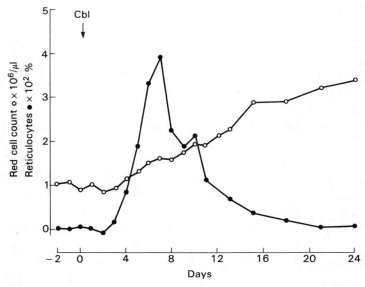

Fig 7.1 In assessing a haematological response to therapy in megaloblastic anaemia the day the haematinic is given is day 0. The peak reticulocyte count is reached on day 5, 6 or 7 (in this patient day 7) and the percentage of reticulocytes relate to the degree of anaemia. In this case the red cell count is $1.0 \times 10^6/\mu l$ and the expected reticulocyte count should be between 36–47%. It is 39%. Finally in an optimum response the red cell count should reach or exceed $3 \times 10^6/\mu l$ in the third week.

63

folate will cause all the early cells to mature in a synchronous manner. Thus there is a synchronous release of new red cells to the blood and these constitute the reticulocyte peak which characterizes the response of a severe megaloblastic anaemia. In an optimal response the reticulocyte peak is reached on day 5, 6 or 7 after the initial dose of treatment which is termed day 0 (Fig. 7.1). The height of the peak is related to the severity of anaemia and may be about 40% when the red cell count is $1-1.5 \times 10^6/\mu l$, about 30% when the count is $1.5-2.0 \times 10^6/\mu l$ and is correspondingly smaller in less anaemic patients. The reticulocytosis is accompanied by a steady rise in the red cell count which should exceed $3.0 \times 10^6/\mu l$ on day 15 but will be correspondingly higher in less anaemic patients. All these three factors must be present in an optimal response.

Although the response is assessed in terms of effects on erythropoiesis, the total white cell count rises to normal in 5–7 days, and the platelet count rises in parallel to the increase in reticulocytes, although the maximum level may not be reached till about 14 days.

The blood film shows the presence of large, very polychromatic erythrocytes 2–3 days after treatment but these disappear a few days, later. There is often a transient appearance of normoblasts (normoblastic crisis) before the reticulocyte peak. Hypersegmented neutrophils decline in numbers after the 10th day and are normal after the 14th day. This implies a new generation of white cells developing from post-treatment haemopoietic stem cells. This too is the time required for the return of a normal oxygen burst and normal capacity to kill ingested bacteria [68].

In the few days after treatment there is an increase in the MCV due to the release of large red cells derived from megaloblasts. These have a very short survival and thereafter the fall in the MCV is biphasic. A relatively sharp initial limb due to shortened survival of pre-treatment erythrocytes and thereafter a flatter component due to a young red cell population. The MCV returns to normal most rapidly in the most anaemic patients as their red cells have the shorter survival (20–30 days) and takes longer in mildly anaemic patients (70 days). A fall in MCV below 80 fl generally indicates shortage of iron and an emergent iron deficiency anaemia.

In the marrow, megaloblasts generally disappear after 36 hours but giant metamyelocytes persist up to 12 days being phagocytosed by macrophages.

The clinical response

The response of a patient with severe pernicious anaemia to treatment is one of the most gratifying phenomena in medicine. Within 1–2 days of treatment there is a return of well being, alertness and appetite. A painful tongue is relieved after 2 days and regeneration of papillae is seen after 4–7 days. Impaired or abnormal tastes disappear over this period. Pyrexia disappears and symptoms such as diarrhoea disappear after 7 days.

Development of neuropathy is arrested. Symptoms of less than 3 months duration usually disappear completely although all cases show improvement. Muscle tenderness, when present, disappears within 1–2 weeks and there is an increase in strength. Sphincter control is soon regained. Mental and psychiatric symptoms too disappear rapidly and hallucinations, confusion, etc. can disappear within a few days. Paraesthesia can disappear in a few weeks but more often there is a slow diminution over months although when they are of long duration mild residual symptoms remain. Severe loss of vibration sense does not recover. Ataxia of short duration too disappears. Lost tendon reflexes return although extensor plantars, when present, persist. About half the patients with visual impairment show an improvement.

The biochemical response

Specific treatment of megaloblastic anaemia reverses the impairment to haemopoiesis and enables virtually all the developing cells in the marrow to mature into erythrocytes and granulocytes. There is thus a fall in bilirubin within a few hours of treatment and ineffective haemopoiesis (the increased early peak of ^{15}N stercobilinogen from ^{15}N glycine) is normalized.

The serum iron falls in the first 24 hours and this is a useful indicator that the patient is going to respond. In a patient with pernicious anaemia given Cbl, the serum folate falls from say 15 ng/ml to 5 ng/ml in 24 hours. Since reticulocytes (and young red cells) have more folate that older cells, red cell folate rises with the reticulocytosis.

Urinary Figlu and urinary MMA excretion fall in the first 2 days and are normal after 5–7 days.

In folate deficiency where the serum Cbl level may be low, there is a rise in the serum Cbl over the first 10 days of folate treatment.

Therapy is accompanied by a strongly positive nitrogen balance. There is an increased excretion of uric acid reaching a maximum on day 4 after treatment. The plasma potassium may fall and in anaemic elderly patients a supplement may be a useful precaution. Whole body potassium increases steadily due to an increase in the red cell mass. Rarely, low potassium is accompanied by lactic acidosis which too responds to treatment for the anaemia. Chromosomal abnormalities disappear. There is a small increase in immunoglobulins.

Abnormal enzyme activities are corrected within 1 to 3 days and these include LDH. Low serum cholesterol has been noted in untreated megaloblastic anaemia and this too is restored within a few days of therapy. In patients with renal failure folic acid lowers the plasma homocysteine level possibly by promoting its remethylation to methionine [69].

The sub-optimal haematological response

Here the reticulocyte peak is far lower than expected from the degree of anaemia, it occurs later than day 7 and there is little if any increase in the red cell count. Occasionally there may even be an apparently good reticulocyte response but this is not accompanied by an adequate rise in the red cell count. Further, the patient does not show any clinical benefit.

If diagnosis is correct an accompanying disorder may have been overlooked. Occult infection as in the respiratory or renal system or active tubercle infection may be present. The patient may also have a second disease such as renal failure, active rheumatoid arthritis, thyrotoxicosis or incipient cardiac failure, which may be the explanation. When the patient is a candidate for anaemia of chronic disorders, treatment of the megaloblastic anaemia may produce a slow rise in red cell count, etc. to the level expected in anaemia of chronic disorders.

Therapy with folate antagonists such as Septrin or Bactrim can abolish a reticulocyte response [70] and the response will be resumed after the drug has been stopped.

An optimal response requires an optimal dose of haematinic. This is not less than 80 µg Cbl as a single dose or not less than 2 µg Cbl daily both by injection. In a patient with normal folate requirements a minimum of 300 µg folate daily is required but in a patient with increased folate requirement such as sickle-cell anaemia, or in pregnancy up to 500 µg folate daily may be required. Liver extracts are no longer used but these often supplied sub-optimal doses of Cbl. Too small a dose may be the explanation for a poor response.

Whereas for all practical purposes patients with folate deficiency do not respond to Cbl, all patients with megaloblastic anaemia respond to folate. The dose of folate needed is probably greater in order to obtain a response in primary Cbl deficiency than it would be in primary folate deficiency. The size of the dose has not been explored in detail. Giving the wrong haematinic is thus another cause for a poor response.

'Non-specific' responses can be obtained in megaloblastic anaemia by a variety of substances that appear able to contribute a 1-carbon unit or bypass a biochemical block. These include histidine, choline, serine, pyrimidine precursors such as carbamylaspartic acid, orotic acid, uridylic acid and cytidylic acid. Thymidine has also given responses.

Steroids and antibiotics such as penicillin and tetracycline have been associated with responses. In these cases the response has generally been a small increase in reticulocytes with little increase in red cell count.

Treatment with both Cbl and folate

Therapy with both these haematinics is not advised. The patient if deficient in either, will respond but little will have been learnt. Nevertheless, in pernicious anaemia administration of Cbl and folate produce extremely good responses and is accompanied by more rapid restoration of normoblastic haemopoiesis than is achieved with a single haematinic [432].

It is rare to find significant deficiency of both Cbl and folate in the same patient. This can only be proven by first treating with Cbl and when the reticulocytes have returned to baseline adding folate when a second reticulocyte response should occur.

Relapse on cessation of therapy

On stopping Cbl injections relapse can occur within months or after years even as many as 20. The time depends on the amount of Cbl received and on the extent of restoration of Cbl stores. Relapse of 41 patients treated with liver injections is shown in Fig. 7.2 [71].

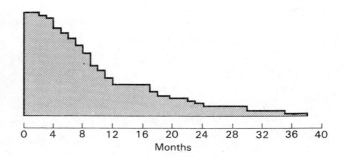

Fig. 7.2 Forty-one patients with pernicious anaemia who were treated by liver injections, stopped treatment and the time before each relapsed is indicated. Most relapsed within a year. Liver extract supplied far smaller amounts of Cbl than is now used in treatment and hence a patient treated with Cbl is likely to remain in remission for years after stopping therapy.

Chapter 8 Biochemical basis of megaloblastic anaemia

Recent years have brought considerable clarification to our understanding of the consequences of deficiency of Cbl and folate. Earlier years were dominated by the methylfolate trap hypothesis formulated in 1962 [72,73]. The transfer of the methyl group of methylfolate to homocysteine to form methionine requires Cbl as coenzyme and this step is considerably impaired in Cbl deficiency (Fig. 8.1, step 2). There is no disagreement with this interpretation.

$$\text{MethyleneH}_4\text{folate} \xrightarrow{\quad 1 \quad} \text{MethylH}_4\text{folate} \xrightarrow[2]{\text{Cbl}} \text{H}_4\text{folate} + \text{methionine}$$

Fig. 8.1 The enzyme methylenetetrahydrofolate reductase converts methyleneH$_4$folate to methylH$_4$folate (1). *In vitro* studies indicate that the reaction favours methylH$_4$folate synthesis and *in vitro* the reaction is unlikely to go to the left to any significant degree. Thus *in vitro* once methylH$_4$folate is formed it is unlikely to be oxidized back to methyleneH$_4$folate. The methyl group of methylH$_4$folate is transferred to homocysteine to form methionine (2) and this step requires cobalamin coenzyme. In Cbl deficiency reaction 2 fails, and as the methyl group cannot be oxidized to methylene, methylH$_4$folate is said to accumulate. If correct, this would result in increasing amounts of folate being immobilized or trapped as methylH$_4$folate.

If the methyl group of methylfolate cannot be disposed of by transfer *in toto*, neither can it be oxidized back to methylene ($-CH_2-$) and formate ($-CHO$). This is because *in vitro* studies show that the thermodynamics of the methylenetetrahydrofolate reductase reaction ($-CH_2 \rightarrow CH_3$) is very strongly to the right (Fig. 8.1, step 1). Thus on this basis in Cbl deficiency there is nowhere for the methyl group to go. As more folate entered the methyl form, so it was increasingly trapped as methylfolate. As formylfolate is needed for purine synthesis and methylenefolate for thymidine synthesis it was postulated that with methylfolate trapping there was insufficient folate left outside the trap to meet the needs for synthesis of these essential nucleotides needed for DNA and RNA synthesis.

The methylene reductase reaction is readily reversed *in vitro* if an electron acceptor is provided, such as menadione. Under these circumstances the methyl group is stoichiometrically converted into methylene. However, the biochemical view was that the mammalian body was unable to provide such an electron acceptor. This interpretation has been shown to be in error. Studies with intact animals have demonstrated that the methyl group is readily oxidized, not only in healthy animals but also in Cbl-deficient animals.

Increasing the dietary content of methionine or giving a parenteral injection of methionine causes a virtual disappearance of methylfolate from liver within minutes. The amount of methionine producing this effect in the intact animal is within the range normally taken in the diet. The disappearance of methylfolate is accompanied by a rise in formylfolate and tetrahydrofolate (Fig. 8.2) as well as by an increase in exhaled CO_2 indicating oxidation of the methyl group. This

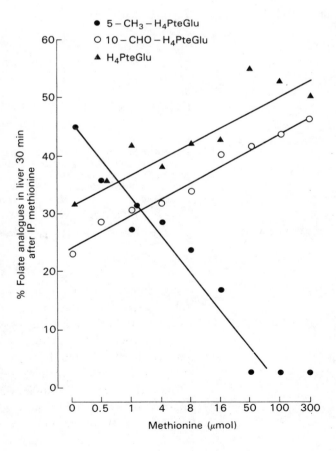

Fig. 8.2 *In vivo* methionine given in physiological doses causes oxidation of methylH$_4$folate (●) to formylH$_4$folate (○) and to H$_4$folate (▲) when the 'C' is oxidized to CO_2. In this study rats were killed 30 min after an injection of methionine and liver folates analysed. About 95% of methylH$_4$folate disappears 30 min after 50 µmol methionine. Thus unlike the *in vitro* situation, in the intact animal the methyl group of methylH$_4$folate is readily oxidized.

occurs in both control and Cbl-deficient animals [74,433]. Even in the absence of added methionine, however, the Cbl-deficient animal oxidizes the methyl group of methylfolate [75] (Fig. 8.3). It does so by using methylfolate as the substrate for synthesizing methylfolatepolyglutamate and when five additional glutamic acid residues have been added to from methylfolatehexaglutamate, the methyl group is oxidized promptly. Thus there is no methylfolate trapping and the Cbl-deficient animal is able to metabolize its methylfolate.

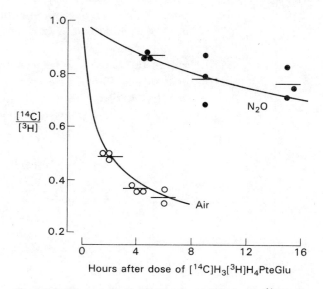

Fig. 8.3 In this study methylH$_4$folate was labelled with [^{14}C] in the methyl group and with [^{3}H] in the pteridine portion. Thus the two parts of the molecule could be followed separately. Further the ratio of [^{14}C] to [^{3}H] was adjusted to unity so that a loss of [^{14}C] would result in a fall of the ratio below 1. Rats were given doubly-labelled methylH$_4$folate, killed at varying times (0.5–16 hours later), liver removed, methylfolate isolated and the ratio of [^{14}C] to [^{3}H] determined. In air breathing rats (○) the half-life of the methyl group was 2 hours. The rate of oxidation of the methyl group was slower in rats in which Cbl had been inactivated by 3 days exposure to N$_2$O (●).

In addition other data are not accounted for by the methylfolate trap. The most important is the failure of the Cbl-deficient animal to use tetrahydrofolate, which is outside the hypothetical trap. Thus the Cbl-deficient animal cannot use tetrahydrofolate for folate polyglutamate formation (Table 8.1), for thymidine synthesis (Fig. 8.4) [76], nor for metabolism of histidine [77]. Similar data are available with human marrow cells (Fig. 8.5). These studies, which have failed to substantiate the methylfolate trap, were able to use a new

Table 8.1 The amount of folate polyglutamate formed in rat liver in the 24 hours after an injection of a labelled folate substrate

Substrate	Percentage of folate substrate in rat liver converted into folate polyglutamate	
	Air breathing	N_2O breathing
PteGlu	51	0
H_4PteGlu	55	0
5–CH_3H_4PteGlu	42	0
10–$CHOH_4$PteGlu	52	46
5,10–$CH=H_4$PteGlu	55	59
5–$CHOH_4$PteGlu	52	49

Air breathing rats converted about half of the six folate analogues into folate polyglutamate (first column). Rats in which Cbl was inactivated by breathing nitrous oxide (N_2O) (second column) were not able to make any folate polyglutamate from the first three substrates and, in particular, could not use tetrahydrofolate (H_4PteGlu) at all. However, they were able to make normal amounts of polyglutamate when folates with a formyl group (CHO–) was supplied as in the last three substrates. This suggests that the effect of Cbl deficiency is due to the failure of formylation of tetrahydrofolate.

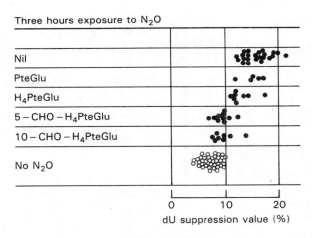

Fig. 8.4 The dU suppression test was carried out on rat marrow cells after 3 hours exposure to N_2O which inactivates Cbl. Normal rat marrow gives a value below 10% (bottom line) and this is always greater than 10% after N_2O (top line). Folic acid and H_4folate (line 2 and 3 from the top) did not improve the result but formylH_4folate (lines 4 and 5) produced a significant correction of thymidine 'synthesis'. Thus the Cbl inactivated rat could not use H_4folate, a finding not predicted by the methylfolate trap but can use formylH_4folate which overcomes the Cbl block.

investigational model, namely, an intact animal exposed to nitrous oxide (N_2O) which totally oxidized and inactivated reduced Cbl. The data that have emerged since 1978 have completely changed our ideas about how Cbl deficiency affects the mammalian organism.

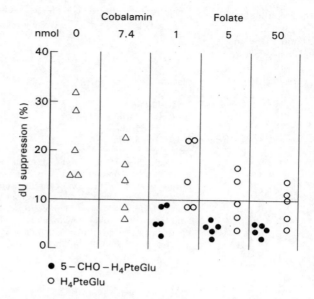

Fig. 8.5 The dU suppression test in five patients with untreated pernicious anaemia. The result was abnormal in all five patients (column 1) and was partially improved by 7.4 nmol of Cbl added to the reaction mixture (column 2). Thereafter H_4folate and CHOH$_4$folate were compared at three dose levels. At all levels formylH$_4$folate was more effective than H_4folate and even 50 nmol of H_4folate (column 5) was less effective than 1 nmol formylH$_4$folate (column 3). Thus in man as in the rat, in Cbl deficiency H_4folate is not used normally and the Cbl block is overcome by formylH$_4$folate.

What causes the megaloblast?

It is likely that the morphological changes seen in the mega-loblast relate to the abnormally slender and elongated chromosomes present in megaloblastic anaemia and to the large number of chromosome breaks that are present [18], that is, it is related to the way formed DNA is assembled within a cell. Hypomethylation inhibits the establishment of DNA supercoils and affects the orientation of DNA helix formation [19]. About 5% of cystosine residue on DNA are normally methylated but, as yet, studies with restriction enzymes specific for methylated cytosine have not provided firm evidence of hypomethylation.

The megaloblast does not arise from lack of nucleosides since these are present in marked excess.

It has to be confessed that we do not have the explanation for the development of the megaloblast. Nor do we know why man uniquely becomes megaloblastic as a result of Cbl deficiency, although Cbl neuropathy can be produced in primates, fruit bats and pigs.

The supply of 1-carbon units

It is the general view that the main source of 1-carbon units for purine and pyrimidine synthesis is the β carbon of the amino acid, serine. When cobalamin is inactivated a series of events occur which have adverse effects on the availability of 1-carbon units and on transmethylation reactions.

Serine is no longer as readily available in the whole Cbl-deficient animal as a source of 1-carbon units as it may be in control animals. Administration of serine fails to influence events in the Cbl-deficient animal whereas other compounds such as methionine, S-adenosylmethionine, methylthiodenosine are all active. As an example, the Cbl-deficient animal shows an impairment in thymidine synthesis. The enzyme thymidylate synthetase is induced and the transhydroxymethylase pathway by which serine donates a 1-carbon unit to form methyleneH₄folate is unaffected by Cbl deficiency. Nevertheless serine does not correct this defect although formyltetrahydrofolate and methionine [78] both do so. If, as seems likely, serine no longer is a major contributor of 1-carbon units in the Cbl-deficient intact animal (not *in vitro* systems) it throws an extra burden on other sources of 1-carbon units. Support for this view comes from the significant rise in plasma serine when Cbl is inactivated [79].

There is a major defect in the formation of formyltetrahydrofolate. The evidence for this is as follows.
1 The defects identified in the Cbl-deficient animal are reversed by supplying formyltetrahydrofolate [76] but not by tetrahydrofolate.
2 Following inactivation of Cbl there is a sustained rise of endogeneous formate in liver, brain and blood.
3 There is increased urinary excretion of formate in Cbl deficiency.
4 The concentration of formylH₄folate falls to very low levels. Tetrahydrofolate is also low although not as low as formylH₄folate.
5 There is induction of the enzyme, formyltetrahydrofolate synthetase which forms formylH₄folate. At the same time there is a marked decline in activity of the enzyme, cyclohydrolase, which reduces the formyl group to methenyl. These changes suggest a response to a shortage of formylH₄folate.

Thus there is a strong suspicion that serine may not be available in Cbl deficiency and that formate is not properly used to form formylH₄folate.

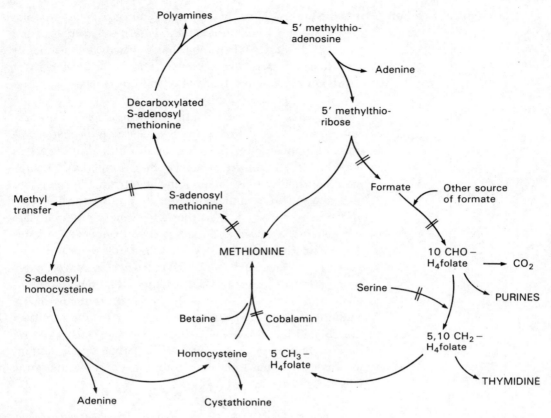

Fig. 8.6 Some pathways involved in Cbl and folate metabolism. The sites where the pathways are diminished or severely curtailed in Cbl deficiency are shown by a double line.

The role of methionine and its derivatives (Fig. 8.6). Not only does formyltetrahydrofolate overcome Cbl-deficiency but it is also reversed by methionine and metabolic products of methionine. Cbl deficiency results in loss of activity of two enzymes, methionine synthetase and methylmalonyl-CoA mutase. In liver there is a second enzyme that can methylate homocysteine to form methionine, betaine homocysteine methyltransferase. This is induced following Cbl inactivation and, in part, compensates for the loss of the Cbl-dependent pathway. This compensation is however incomplete because the level of S-adenosylmethionine continues to decline. Methionine is an important donor of 1-carbon units. Not only can the methyl group of methionine be oxidized to methylene, formate and CO_2 [80] but an active formate unit is released through a pathway involved in polyamine synthesis. A product of this pathway is 5'-methylthioribose. Methylthioribose is converted back to methionine and a mole of formate is released for each mole of methionine regenerated. Using methylthioribose appropriately labelled with ^{14}C substantial transfer of this 1-carbon to adenine and guanine has been demonstrated. Harvey Mudd (personal communication) has estimated that the polyamine pathway through which methylthioribose is formed may supply 0.5–1 mmol of formate which is enough to meet man's requirements. Thus reduction in supply of methionine restricts the pathway through methylthioribose and when taken with failure of formylH$_4$-folate synthesis and serine unavailability, indicates an overall lack of 1-carbon units. Reduction of 1-carbon unit supply impairs synthesis of thymidine (abnormal dU suppression test) and impairs purine synthesis. The lack of methionine and hence reduced levels of S-adenosylmethionine account for impaired transmethylation reactions readily demonstrated in reduced ^{14}C transfer into phosphatidylcholine, etc.

Are there other pathways impaired in Cbl deficiency?

There is suggestive evidence that there may be an impairment of transport of metabolites across cell membranes in Cbl deficiency. The failure for serine to influence events and the rise in plasma serine in the Cbl-deficient animal has been discussed. When Cbl is inactivated there is an abrupt rise in plasma methylfolate. One explanation put forward for this is that there is failure to retain methylfolate in cells. For methylfolate to be retained it must be converted into a folatepolyglutamate. In the normal cell it would require transfer of the methyl group and glutamic acid residues added to either H$_4$PteGlu or CHOH$_4$PteGlu. In the Cbl-deficient cell methylfolate itself is used for the addition of glutamic acid residues [75]. As this occurs at a much slower rate than with other substrates (Fig. 8.3) it allows methylfolate to efflux. This explanation is less convincing with isolated cells from patients with untreated pernicious anaemia where there is impaired 'uptake' of methylH$_4$folate [81,82].

When marrow cells are incubated with appropriate 1- carbon units those from Cbl-deficient patients show impaired incorporation into thymidine, choline, etc. Since none of these pathways require Cbl as a coenzyme and the addition of 1-carbon units reverses the failure of supply of these units, an impaired transport into the cell may be an explanation. More definitive studies using isolated cell membranes are required.

The development of Cbl neuropathy

As with methionine synthetase elsewhere, that in brain is also inactivated by N_2O [83] and by Cbl deficiency. This results in a failure to convert homocysteine to methionine. Thus the requirement for methionine in the CNS has to be met by increased transport into the CSF. This has been demonstrated using ^{35}S-methionine in Cbl-inactivated rats (unpublished observations). There is thus a continued entry of methionine into the CNS without an adequate mechanism for the disposal of the end products of its metabolism. S-adenosylmethionine levels can increase above the normal level in Cbl-inactivated animals [84] and increased levels of S-adenosylhomocysteine and cystathionine have been found [85]. However, Cbl neuropathy in fruit bats develops in the absence of any accumulation of homocysteine. It is likely, though not yet shown, that the same defects demonstrated in liver and bone marrow are also present in the CNS and are the cause of Cbl neuropathy.

Primary folate deficiency

The pathogenesis of primary folate deficiency appears to be relatively uncomplicated. There is tissue depletion of folate and hence curtailment of 1-carbon unit transfers to a point where haemopoiesis is abnormal and megaloblastosis ensues.

Chapter 9 Investigation, management and treatment in megaloblastic anaemia

The diagnosis of megaloblastic anaemia and the steps that help to establish whether the cause is Cbl or folate deficiency have been set out earlier in this monograph.

Diagnosis of Cbl deficiency

Cbl deficiency is associated with the following.
Low serum Cbl level.
Generally normal serum folate but not uncommonly low red cell folate.
Increased urinary and plasma methylmalonic acid.
Abnormal dU suppression test partially corrected by the addition of Cbl.
Impaired Cbl absorption except in dietary Cbl deficiency.
Haematological and clinical response to Cbl.

Diagnosis of folate deficiency

Folate deficiency is associated with the following.
Low red cell and serum folate.
Generally normal but not uncommonly low Cbl level.
Normal Cbl absorption.
Increased urinary formiminoglutamic acid excretion.
Abnormal dU suppression not corrected by Cbl.
Haematological and clinical response to folate.

In both Cbl and folate deficiency the disorder producing this deficiency must also be diagnosed. These disorders are listed below.

Causes of Cbl deficiency

Dietary deficiency

Strict vegetarians such as Hindus.
Neonates born to mothers with untreated Cbl deficiency.

Gastric causes

Pernicious anaemia.
Post-gastrectcomy.
Congenital absence or abnormal intrinsic factor.
Destruction of gastric mucosa by a caustic substance.

Intestinal causes   Anatomical abnormalities of the small gut including blind
            loops, strictures, fistulae, small gut diverticulitis, poorly
            functioning gastroenterostomy, Whipple's disease, sclero-
            derma, gut resection.
            Abnormal gut flora.
            Hypogammaglobulinaemia and all the above disorders.
            Diphyllobothrium latum (fish tapeworm) infestation.
            Congenital Cbl malabsorption (Imerslund-Gräsbeck).

Transport defects   Transcobalamin II deficiency.

Metabolic defects   Impairments of cellular metabolism of Cbl.
            Chronic nitrous oxide addiction.

**Causes of folate
deficiency**
Dietary deficiency   Indequate amounts of poor quality food which may be
            associated with alcoholism and scurvy.
Intestinal causes   Gluten-sensitive enteropathy.
            Tropical sprue.
            Congenital folate malabsorption.

Increased folate   Pregnancy.
requirement   Chronic haemolytic anaemia including haemoglobinopathy
            and malaria, exfoliative skin disorders, chronic myelofibrosis.

Drugs   Folate antagonists including methotrexate, pyrimethamine,
            trimethoprim, triamterene, salazopyrene.

**Treatment in
megaloblastic anaemia**
Blood transfusion   Transfusion should only be considered in very anaemic
            patients who are suffering severe effects from anaemia includ-
            ing cardiac failure, severe dyspnoea and angina. It is just in
            such patients that the risk of overloading the circulation is
            greatest and where transfusion can have a fatal outcome.
            Wherever possible, having collected the appropriate samples
            and obtained a marrow, the effects of both Cbl and folate
            given together, should be tried. If there is no improvement in
            36 hours, it may be necessary to give 1 unit of packed red cells
            slowly over 6 hours combined with a diuretic. The patient
            should be propped up in bed, kept warm and observed care-
            fully. Evidence of circulatory overload is a rise in venous
            pressure, restlessness, a dry cough and moist sounds at the

lung bases. If this happens, 100 ml of blood should be removed from the other arm and if a diuresis has not been obtained, a further intravenous diuretic given. Mortality among anaemic patients treated in this way can be as high as 14% [86]

Specific therapy

It is a general principal that, except in the extreme situation outlined above, only one haematinic should be given and sufficient time allowed to demonstrate its effect. In this way information as to the underlying deficiency is obtained. The clinical situation will determine which haematinic should be given first and should data become available indicating the choice was incorrect, a more appropriate haematinic can be added. Generally, 7–10 days is required to assess a response.

Cobalamin therapy

Both hydroxocobalamin (OHCbl) and cyanocobalamin (CNCbl) are available and methylcobalamin has been used particularly in Japan. Generally the doses used in treatment have been large and more than enough to achieve all the objectives of a reasonable treatment schedule. In the treatment of Cbl deficiency the initial objective is to obtain an optimal haematological and clinical response including maximal restoration of CNS damage and thereafter to maintain optimal Cbl stores.

The treatment of dietary deficiency should ideally be a broadening of the diet to include foods of animal origin. This may well be unacceptable to many lifelong vegetarians, particularly elderly subjects. In these a daily oral Cbl supplement is advised and this should be not less than 5 µg Cbl daily. Some foods such as some cereals have a Cbl supplement added and this too, if taken regularly, can be an important source of Cbl.

Apart from dietary Cbl deficiency, deficiency always arises from impaired Cbl absorption and thus parenteral administration of Cbl is necessary. Other methods of administration are available.

Two advantages have been claimed for the use of OHCbl as the preferred form of Cbl in clinical practice. Firstly, it is better retained by the body. Table 9.1 shows that there is a significantly smaller loss of OHCbl into the urine than there is with an equivalent injection of CNCbl. This seems to be a sensible reason for using OHCbl. OHCbl possibly disperses more slowly from an injection site and binds more strongly to plasma proteins such as albumin. Correspondingly plasma Cbl levels in pernicious anaemia remained elevated for a

Table 9.1 Urinary loss of Cbl following parenteral injection (% of dose)

Dose (μg)	OHCbl	CNCbl
100	8	45
500	25	70
1000	29	85

longer period after OHCbl than after CNCbl. Thus with a 500 μg dose the plasma Cbl level remained above 100 pg/ml in pernicious anaemia on average for 289 days with OHCbl and for 114 days with CNCbl [87]. Individual patient variation was considerable. Thus with 100 μg CNCbl by injection the plasma Cbl level fell below 200 pg/ml after 1–6 weeks and with OHCbl in 4–10 weeks.

Two further reasons have been given for preferring OHCbl: that the cyanide moiety of CNCbl is toxic and that CNCbl is of no use in treating optic neuritis (tobacco amblyopia). Suggestions that Cbl can be inactivated by excess cyanide or cyanide-containing foods have not been supported by any evidence. CNCbl, other than a possible trace component in plasma, has not been identified in tissues. Claims that optic neuritis has to be treated with OHCbl are based on a limited uncontrolled study in a few patients [88]. Others have taken the view that a significant proportion of such patients recover irrespective of the manner of treatment and that Cbl has no special role in the treatment of tobacco amblyopia.

Treatment should allow the retention of about 2 μg Cbl daily. OHCbl as 250 μg every 4 or 8 weeks meets this requirement. In the initial stages of treatment it is usual to give such a dose daily or on alternate days for say 5–6 doses in order to replenish Cbl stores. Whether this actually happens is not known. Since all these doses are larger than required for a maximal response (? one dose of 80 μg) it is not of great moment. There is no evidence that patients with neuropathy require larger doses; indeed, a regimen that produces restoration of the blood will also, in time, produce the greatest recovery of the nervous system.

About 1% of an oral dose of Cbl is absorbed in pernicious anaemia presumably by passive diffusion. Thus 200 μg by mouth daily will allow about 2 μg to be absorbed and 1000 μg about 10 μg. This is a practical approach in the rare situation where the patient is intolerant to injected Cbl.

Cbl has also been absorbed by inhalation and through an aerosol. The addition of IF will allow oral absorption of small doses of Cbl but as the source of IF has been hog's stomach, antibodies formed against the hog material has made this approach impracticable in most patients. Indeed such patients have relapsed with both megaloblastic anaemia and neuropathy. There is no place for slow-release depot preparations of Cbl.

Reactions to Cbl   Allergic and anaphylactic reactions to Cbl are rare and recur with each injection. Urticaria is prominent. A positive response follows intradermal testing with Cbl. Some such patients can be managed by substituting daily oral therapy.

Folate therapy   The pharmacological analogue, pteroylglutamic acid, is available as 5 mg tablets. 5-Formyltetrahydropteroylglutamic acid (folinic acid, leucovorin factor) as the D, L mixture is available both as a solution and as tablets. Only the L isomer is biologically active. Folinic acid is used primarily to limit toxicity of folate antagonists such as methotrexate.

As the folate content of the liver in a healthy adult averages 10 mg and a similar amount may be present in the rest of the

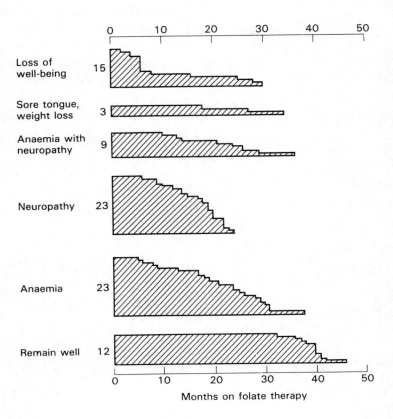

Fig. 9.1 Eighty-five patients in whom pernicious anaemia had been diagnosed, were treated with 5 mg folic acid daily. Fifteen stopped treatment because they had felt better while on an earlier liver injection regimen. Three had a sore tongue, 23 developed neuropathy and 23 anaemia which was megaloblastic in those in whom marrow aspiration was performed and 9 relapsed with both anaemia and neuropathy. Twelve remained well; perhaps these did not have pernicious anaemia [71].

body, daily folate doses of 5–15 mg daily are clearly very large. After the first dose the bulk is excreted in the urine. Five mg pteroylglutamic acid once daily is adequate therapy. Unless given prophylactically to patients with permanently high folate requirements such as those with sickle-cell anaemia and chronic myelofibrosis, therapy is usually given for about 4 weeks.

Folic acid is generally free of side effects. Rarely an individual can be sensitized to a dose and a second exposure produces a generalized pruritic erythematous skin reaction, malaise and bronchospasm. Intradermal tests with folic acid give large wheals but results are negative with folinic acid. In animals very large doses of folate produce precipitation of folic acid in the renal tubules and renal tubular necrosis.

Long-term folate has been found by some to aggravate fit frequency in epileptics and rarely a single dose of folate may precipitate status epilepticus [89, 90]. Long-term folate is also contraindicated in patients with pernicious anaemia not receiving Cbl since it can precipitate neuropathy, anaemia and glossitis. Figure 9.1 shows the results among 85 patients diagnosed as having pernicious anaemia given folic 5 mg daily [71]. The vast majority relapse either with anaemia, neuropathy or both. In some, relapse, particularly with neuropathy, can be relatively acute. The diagnosis of pernicious anaemia must be questioned in those who remain in remission.

Chapter 10   Pernicious anaemia

Pernicious anaemia (PA) is a disorder in which there is megaloblastic haemopoiesis and/or a neuropathy due to Cbl deficiency, the result of Cbl malabsorption due to severe atrophic gastritis.

History   It is not certain to whom to attribute the first description of PA [7]. An account of a patient with numbness of fingers, hands and forearms, macrocytosis and gastric atrophy by Osler and Gardner in 1877 [91] qualifies. It is possible that Combe in Edinburgh in 1822 and Addison in London in 1855 described patients who might have had PA, as did Handfield-Jones in 1853 and Biermer in 1872. Gastric atrophy was described by Fenwick in 1870 and was followed by the finding of achlorhydria by Cahn and Von Mehring in 1886. Paul Ehrlich in 1880 described megaloblasts in the marrow. Spinal cord involvement was recognized by Lichtheim in 1887. The clinical picture of Cbl neuropathy was described by Russell, Batten and Collier in 1900. Finally in 1926 Minot and Murphy demonstrated the beneficial effect of liver and this led to the isolation of Cbl 20 years later by the Merck team in the USA and the Glaxo team in the UK.

Occurrence   A survey of 16 million people registered with doctors in the UK gave a frequency of PA of 127 for 100 000 population [92]. Similar frequencies have been noted in Denmark and Sweden. Adequate data are not available elsewhere. A survey among a population of Indians from Gujerat living in London suggested a frequency of not less than 128 per 100 000 [16]. Many case reports of PA among patients of African descent have appeared in recent years. No race is immune even if the frequency remains to be determined.

The frequency among women consistently outnumbers men, the female to male ratio being 10 to 7. It is a disease of later life and only 11% of patients present before the age of 40. Over the age of 60 the frequency of PA approaches 1%, 2.5% over the age of 65 in Glasgow and 3.7% over the age of 75 in North-West England [7]. Where there is a family history of PA or autoimmune disease the mean age at diagnosis was 51 years as compared to 66 in the absence of such a history [93] and where several autoimmune disorders co-exist, PA can present in the second decade.

Clinical presentation

The presenting features, symptoms and signs that occur in untreated patients have been discussed in Chapter 2. Not uncommonly these features are modified by accompanying disorders that are discussed below.

Natural history of pernicious anaemia

Before the advent of effective therapy some 60 years ago, PA was uniformly fatal. Expectation of life was generally less than 3 years from the time of diagnosis and survival for longer than 5 years was unusual. Nevertheless, it was usual for spontaneous remissions to occur with a rise in red cell count and clinical improvement which lasted for several months and in some for as long as a year. Second remissions were not uncommon. There was no relief from the neuropathy however and the patients finally lapsed into lethargy, coma and death. With hindsight a meal supplying an adequate dose of folate might have been responsible for these remissions.

With treatment the survival in women is the same as that of the general population but there is a higher mortality in males, possibly due to gastric neoplasms.

Aetiology and pathogenesis
Stomach

'I suspect that in these cases [PA] there exists degenerative disease of the glandular tubules of the stomach' (Austin Flint 1860). The site of the primary lesion in PA indeed is the stomach. Atrophy of the body of the stomach is present in all patients. The wall is reduced to about one-half or less of normal thickness and there is an abrupt demarcation at the relatively normal antrum. All the coats are affected. The columns of secreting tubules of parietal and oxyntic cells disappear and are replaced by a mucus-producing mucosa often of intestinal type (intestinal metaplasia). There is considerable infiltration by lymphocytes and plasma cells. *Campylobacter pyloridis* is absent in what has been termed type A gastritis. The outer muscle coats are similarly atrophic.

In up to one-third of patients, however, small numbers of parietal cells persist and these remain functional producing very small amounts of intrinsic factor and even trace amounts of hydrochloric acid.

As a result of this very severe loss of secretory cells, there is a marked reduction in the output of gastric juice. Control subjects secrete between 50 and 150 ml gastric juice over 1 hour; in PA this is only 15–20 ml. Furthermore, a stimulant to gastric secretion such as gastrin or its analogues produces a large increase in gastric secretion in healthy subjects but there is none in PA.

It is unusual for the pH of the stimulated gastric secretion to be below 6.0 in PA and more usually the pH is alkaline. Very rarely the pH can be as low as 4. Pepsinogen activity is absent. Two-thirds of patients with PA have no detectable IF in the gastric juice and one-third secrete less than 200 units IF in 1 hour [94]. Generally the concentration of IF, when present, was less than 6 units/ml but one patient secreted 11 units/ml after histamine stimulation (Fig. 4.2). R-binders are present in normal amount in PA gastric juice samples and these are not diluted in the post-stimulation gastric juice as there is no increase in volume of secretion.

These findings are not unique to PA. They can also be found in severe simple atrophic gastritis. The PA patient differs in two respects, the presence of megaloblastic haemopoiesis and/or neuropathy and the presence of humoral and cell-mediated immunity to intrinsic factor.

Radiologically the PA stomach shows a loss of rugal markings and hypotonicity [95]. Gastric endoscopy may reveal a recognizable atrophic mucosa. In addition it reveals a high incidence of polyps, small carcinoid tumours and carcinoma in patients with PA.

Atrophic gastritis leads to hyperplasia of endocrine cells in the antral mucosa. Very high serum gastrin levels are the rule in PA (mean of 1000 and 200 pg/ml in PA and control sera, respectively). Food is the stimulus to gastrin release and the acid produced thereafter is the feedback control that halts gastrin production. Achlorhydria results in loss of feedback inhibition and is accompanied by proliferation of gastric enterochromaffin-like cells. Their secretions include in addition to gastrin, 5-hydroxytryptamine, vasoactive intestinal polypeptide and substance P [96]. Of 30 cases of gastric carcinoid at the Mayo clinic, 12 had PA [97]. Endoscopy performed in 123 PA patients showed that, in addition to an increase in endocrine cells, four had solitary and one had multiple endocrine tumours [98]. These carcinoid tumours may be small and only be detected microscopically when multiple biopsies are taken; in others they appear as small orange spots about 2 mm in diameter with dilated irregular capillaries as well as macroscopic lesions or polyps. Among 71 PA patients followed for an average of 7 years, carcinoids were present in 4% and gastric carcinoma in 3% [99]. The very small carcinoids appear to carry little risk of malignant transformation and are not associated with clinical manifestations of the carcinoid syndrome. Larger carcinoids do carry a risk of malignant change and clinical symptoms.

A further hazard for patients with PA as well as patients with atrophic gastritis without PA is carcinoma of the stomach. Follow-up of 658 patients with PA seen in Boston between 1915 and 1951 showed that between 5 and 8% died with a gastric carcinoma [100]. In 1986 Borch [101] reported five malignant carcinoid tumours and five adenocarcinomas among 123 PA patients. All these were diagnosed on initial clinical presentation and no new ones appeared on follow-up.

Varis [102] estimates that in the Finnish population over the age of 65 years, 43% have atrophic gastritis of the body of the stomach and 6% have severe atrophic gastritis. PA is present in 0.72% and gastric cancer in 0.32%. Of new gastric cancers only a few are associated with PA. It was calculated that the annual incidence of gastric cancer in PA is 0.3%; this is three times higher than that in the general population.

Autoimmunity   There is general agreement that both the development of gastric atrophy and ultimate failure of IF secretion is the result of autoimmune factors. Patients with PA have humoral antibodies against both the gastric parietal cell and IF and cell-mediated immunity against IF. There are alterations to T cell subsets that too may be relevant.

Antibodies reacting with parietal cells are present in sera of about 90% of patients with PA as well as in up to 16% of control sera. Reaction may be with part of the parietal-cell membrane, with gastrin receptors and some antibodies may be cytotoxic. The administration of parietal-cell antibodies to rats produced mild atrophic changes and a marked decline in acid secretion [103]. Parietal-cell antibodies are also present in most gastric-juice samples from PA patients.

Antibodies against IF were present in 54% of 882 sera from PA patients. These antibodies react with the site on the IF molecule binding Cbl and hence prevent Cbl absorption. Some sera, in addition, react with the IF–Cbl complex. Possibly they may prevent IF–Cbl attachment to the ileal-binding site. IF antibodies are relatively unique to PA. Rarely they may be found in sera from patients with Graves' disease, and relatives of patients with PA [46]. IF antibodies also occur in the gastric juice in PA when they are usually IgA immuno-globulins. The serum antibody is usually IgG. In gastric juice the antibody is usually present as an IF–antibody complex.

In addition to humoral antibody in sera and gastric juice, cell-mediated immunity directed against IF can be demon-strated in 86% of PA patients [45], including those patients with hypogammaglobulinaemia (who cannot make humoral antibody) and PA. Humoral and/or cell-mediated immunity against IF was present in 24 out of 25 patients with PA in whom all the investigations were performed [45].

There is a considerable increase in the numbers of IgA-secreting lymphocytes in the gastric mucosa in PA and a smaller increase in IgG-secreting lymphocytes [105]. In addi-tion marked increases in T-lymphocytes have been found [106].

Circulating T-cell subsets have been assessed in treated PA patients. These show a significant fall in the numbers of T-suppressor cells in PA patients who have IF antibodies [107]. The decline in T-suppressor cell activity may allow the devel-opment of lymphoid clones against IF and parietal cells in-cluding specific cytoxic killer cells that lead to loss of gastric-secreting cells. These changes can be reversed by treating PA patients with steroids. Under these circumstances there is a recovery in Cbl absorption, a re-appearance of new parietal cells on gastric biopsy and a return of some hydrochloric acid and IF in the gastric secretion [108].There is a fall in the level of humoral IF antibody but the improvement in Cbl absorp-tion is an early event suggesting an effect of steroids in rever-sing local immune factors in the GI tract. The benefits are lost after steroid withdrawal.

Clinical associations with pernicious anaemia

A variety of disorders occur with greater frequency in patients who have PA and among family of PA patients. These are autoimmune disorders and when such disorders co-exist the clinical presentation may be altered.

In addition other blood disorders like polycythaemia rarely and thalassaemia frequently co-exist with PA and cause problems not only in diagnosis but in management.

Familial incidence of pernicious anaemia

It is common for one or more additional cases of PA to be present among a patients' family. This is so in about 20% of patients in the UK and in about 30% of cases in Denmark. The frequency of PA among first and second degree relatives is 2.5% as compared to a frequency of 0.13% among a control group [109]. Concordance is present in most cases of identical twins with PA. However, when both parents have PA, the tendency of the offspring to get PA is no greater than when only one parent or a family member has PA. Among family members of PA probands some 24% have parietal-cell antibodies indicating the likelihood of autoimmune gastritis.

There is a slight excess of blood group A among PA patients as well as among patients with carcinoma of the stomach.

The association of PA with human leukocyte antigens (HLA) is less strong than for other autoimmune disorders. HLA-B8 is strongly linked with autoimmune disease, particularly in the polyendocrinopathy syndrome. Patients with endocrine disease and PA are associated with HLA-B8, B15 and B18. There is stronger association with the HLA-DR2 allele and possibly with DR5 [110–112]. The variable reports of association or lack of it in the literature reflect the small number of patients in such studies.

Thyroid and other endocrine disease

The strongest clinical association of PA is with primary myxoedema. Thus some 9% of patients with myxoedema also have PA. The association is less strong with hyperthyroidism, 2.4% of whom also have PA. Follow-up of patients with PA requires regular assessment of thyroid function, preferably by estimation of the level of thyroid stimulating hormone (TSH). Among over 5800 patients with PA selected from the literature,

Table 10.1 The frequency of parietal-cell and thyroid antibodies in PA, autoimmune disorders and their relatives

Disorder	Frequency of:	
	Parietal-cell antibodies (%)	Thyroid antibodies (%)
PA	84	55
PA relatives	36	50
Myxoedema	32	87
Graves' disease	28	53
'Thyroid disease' relatives	20	46
Iron-deficiency anaemia	24	—
Iron-deficiency relatives	8	—
Adrenal atrophy	23	31
Controls	0–16	0–15

1.8% had Graves' disease and 2.4% myxoedema. The latter figure suggests underdiagnosis.

There is also an association between PA and idiopathic adrenal failure, hypoparathyroidism and premature ovarian failure. Table 10.1 shows the frequency of parietal-cell and thyroid antibodies in these disorders. Alopecia and vitiligo too tend to be associated with these autoimmune disorders.

The association of PA and diabetes mellitus is a weak one. Some 2.4% of 5627 PA patients had diabetes which is marginally greater than the incidence in the general population (1.7%). There is a small increase in the frequency of autoantibodies among younger insulin-sensitive diabetics [7].

The autoimmune polyglandular deficiency syndrome

Pernicious anaemia may be part of a familial disorder in which there is multiple failure of endocrine organs.

Type I presenting in the second decade of life is characterized by the association of hypoparathyroidism, primary adrenal insufficiency (Addison's disease) and mucocutaneous candidiasis. In addition alopecia, PA, intestinal malabsorption, gonadal failure and chronic active hepatitis may occur. The inheritance is possibly autosomal recessive and the different disorders appear at several years interval, starting at about 12 years of age. There is no clear association with HLA alleles [113].

Type II presents at a somewhat later age (30 years) with Addison's disease, thyroid disease and/or insulin-sensitive diabetes mellitus (Schmidt's syndrome). Inheritance is possibly autosomal dominant and there is a linkage with HLA-B8. Vitiligo, PA and gonadal failure also occur [114]. Primary involvement of the pituitary gland leading to gonadal failure may occur [115]. Overt or occult disease may be present in other siblings and there is a need to screen the family.

Over 80% of patients have humoral antibodies against several endocrine glands. There is impaired suppressor T cell function and defective cell-mediated immunity demonstrated against candida in the type I group. Apart from the clinical interest, this group is an example of an association between a defect in cell-mediated immunity, impaired suppressor T cell function and vigorous humoral autoantibody production leading to PA.

Acquired hypogammaglobulinaemia

About 40% of patients with acquired hypogammaglobulinaemia also have PA (12 out of 31 patients) [7]. Diagnosis of PA may be complicated because Cbl malabsorption can be due to giardiasis or an abnormal intestinal flora in these patients. The age of onset is generally the third or fourth decade with a range from 15 to 54 [116]. The PA differs in that not only is the body of the stomach atrophic but the antrum undergoes atrophy as well. As a result these patients, unlike classical PA, have normal serum gastrin levels.

Because these patients are unable to make humoral antibodies, parietal-cell and IF antibodies are absent, the exception being a few patients with immunoglobulin A (IgA) deficiency. However, unlike the polyglandular syndrome, cell-mediated immunity against IF is present and is the reason for the development of PA. There are thus different immune pathways each of which can result in damage to the end organ, in PA, the stomach.

Pure red cell aplasia

At least six examples of PA in association with pure red cell aplasia suggest a significant association. Pure red cell aplasia results from immune suppression of erythroblast formation demonstrable *in vitro* and responds to immune suppression by steroids [7]. Pure red cell aplasia also occurs in patients with the polyglandular deficiency syndrome [117].

Haematological disorders
Iron-deficiency anaemia

Some aspects of iron metabolism in PA have been discussed in Chapter 2. There is some evidence, however, that long-standing iron deficiency may be a contributory factor to the development of PA. This comes from a long-term follow-up of 378 patients who had an iron-deficiency anaemia. Twenty (5.4%) had developed PA and this is a higher frequency than expected [118]. Almost 80% of gastric biopsies from iron-deficient patients show gastritis which is not improved by iron therapy and parietal-cell antibodies are present in 24% of iron-deficient patients. Iron deficiency is accompanied by impaired cell-mediated immunity [119].

Thalassaemia

The simultaneous occurrence of PA (or other megaloblastic anaemia) with either α or β thalassaemia trait can cause confusion in diagnosis. Since red cells in megaloblastic anaemia are macrocytic and those in thalassaemia microcytic, the MCV, when both are present, is usually normal. If anaemia is severe, however, many fragmented red cells may be present and neutrophils are hypersegmented. Treatment of the megaloblastic anaemia causes a fall of the MCV into the range appropriate for thalassaemia.

Iron deficiency and anaemia of chronic disorders, both of which produce small red cells, have the same effect as thalassaemia. In addition the presence of a disorder producing anaemia of chronic disorders may prevent the appearance of a reticulocytosis following treatment and the haemoglobin concentration may slowly drift up to the level determined by the underlying disorder.

Polycythaemia rubra vera   The chance association of PA and polycythaemia can produce some problems in management. Generally such patients present with PA but treatment with Cbl is followed by a very vigorous response with development of polycythaemic blood values within a few months. In a few, pre-existing polycythaemia is complicated by PA with a fall in values and macrocytosis. Each disorder should be treated separately. Cbl in full dose is needed for treating PA and polycythaemia is managed by whatever method is appropriate, bearing in mind the patient's age, etc. It is quite wrong to attempt to give small doses of Cbl that do not permit the haemoglobin to rise to polycythaemic levels. This approach maintains a megaloblastic form of haemopoiesis in order to control the polycythaemia. It has been known to precipitate Cbl neuropathy [7].

Chronic myelofibrosis can also co-exist with PA [7].

Diagnosis   Diagnosis of PA requires the demonstration of the following.
1 Megaloblastic haemopoiesis and/or an appropriate neuropathy.
2 Cbl deficiency.
3 Lack of IF due to gastric atrophy. The way this is done is described in Chapter 4.

Management   Treatment with OHCbl is required for the rest of the patient's life and this is discussed in Chapter 9. Some medical surveillance is desirable in the short-term but thereafter an annual blood count, erythrocyte sedimentation rate (ESR) and TSH level is desirable as routine practice.

In the short-term a significant proportion of treated patients become iron deficient a few months after initiation of therapy. It is rare to have iron deficiency on initial presentation; indeed abundant stainable marrow iron is the rule. But up to 20% of patients run out of iron within a few months of starting Cbl therapy and some after a much longer period [120, 121]. This is detected by a fall in the MCV below the lower limit of 80 fl and thereafter a fall in haemoglobin concentration. However, the late development of iron deficiency is more likely to be due to a bleeding polyp or an intestinal neoplasm and requires appropriate investigation.

It is difficult to justify regular endoscopies in PA to detect early carcinoma as this remains a relatively uncommon complication and the population affected is elderly. An annual check should include a check of weight and ESR and further investigation should only be dictated by clinical circumstances.

However, hypothyroidism is a relatively common complication and measurement of the level of TSH should be done annually.

Chapter 11   Megaloblastic anaemia after gastric surgery

Total gastrectomy

Since total gastrectomy removes all the IF-secreting cells, IF-mediated Cbl absorption ceases. All patients undergoing a total gastrectomy who survive a sufficient length of time and are not given prophylactic Cbl, develop a megaloblastic anaemia due to Cbl deficiency and some develop a neuropathy [7]. Megaloblastic anaemia has been recorded as early as 2 years and as late as 10 years after the operation, the peak being about 5 years later. The period largely relates to the size of Cbl stores.

These patients fail to absorb Cbl given alone, there is generally an improvement when the test is repeated with IF and often there is further improvement in absorption of Cbl–IF after wide spectrum antibiotics such as neomycin, suggesting an abnormal gut flora [122]. Although serum Cbl levels may be maintained for up to 4 months after operation, they then fall rapidly over the subsequent 5–6 months and then decline more slowly to below the normal range.

Prophylactic Cbl has to be started after surgery and continued for life.

Partial gastrectomy

Patients who have undergone a partial gastrectomy are nowadays only found with any frequency among the elderly. Thus in 1982 in Gothenburg, Sweden, some 10% of men among the 70- to 75-year-old age group had undergone a partial gastrectomy for peptic ulceration [123].

Anaemia is common after partial gastrectomy and was present in 28.8% of 7222 patients [7]. This is usually due to iron deficiency, the result of poor absorption of food iron. Megaloblastic anaemia due to Cbl deficiency develops in about 4% of patients after partial gastrectomy. Rarely the megaloblastic anaemia is due to folate deficiency. For all practical purposes, megaloblastic anaemia never appears in under 5 years after an operation removing about 75% of the body of the stomach, although in some it may be delayed for 25 years or more.

93

Not only do these patients have the signs and symptoms of anaemia, but to this is often added the post-prandial symptoms frequent after partial gastrectomy such as a sensation of epigastric fullness, nausea, vomiting, weakness, tremulousness, palpitations, giddiness and syncope. All these symptoms are ameliorated by adequate treatment of the anaemia.

Cbl absorption

Malabsorption of Cbl is only likely when there is loss of IF-secreting (parietal) cells from the gastric remnant. In time atrophic gastritis is present in the gastric remnant after partial gastrectomy in 98% of patients and intestinal metaplasia in 44% [124]. Although only about 4–5% of patients get a megaloblastic anaemia, malabsorption of Cbl is present in between 32 and 43% of patients in different series [7]. However, patients with partial gastrectomy are unusual in so far as Cbl absorption may be improved significantly when a stimulant to gastric (and IF) secretion is given. This can be a meal or an injection of histamine. Thus in two groups of 14 patients the mean urinary excretion of labelled-Cbl in an absorption test was 5.2 and 3.9% of the oral dose which increased to 11.7 and 10.3% respectively when Cbl was given in a meal [125].

Malabsorption of Cbl is more frequent in those patients operated on for a gastric ulcer than a duodenal ulcer [126]. The type of operation does not make a significant difference but the amount of stomach removed is important. The degree of malabsorption of Cbl in those who develop megaloblastic anaemia is not as severe as in pernicious anaemia. Gastrectomy patients generally absorb about twice as much Cbl (0.2 µg of a 1.0 µg dose) as compared to pernicious anaemia patient (0.1 µg of a 1.0 µg dose) presumably because IF-antibodies are present in pernicious anaemia.

In the majority of patients Cbl absorption is improved by the addition of IF (157 out of 178 patients). In those who do not absorb Cbl–IF an abnormal intestinal flora particularly when associated with a blind loop of a polya gastrectomy, is the explanation. On the other hand those patients who have either HCl present in the gastric secretion or a concentration of more than 10 IF units/ml have normal Cbl absorption.

Serum Cbl concentration

Although a recent study failed to find any low Cbl levels after Billroth II resections for duodenal ulcer [127], the accumulated experience in eight series comprising 1274 patients showed that 22% have low Cbl levels [7]. Some 2% of patients have low Cbl levels at 2 years, 9% at 6 years and 14% at 8 years. Low levels are twice as frequent after surgery in gastric as compared to duodenal ulcer patients; and twice as frequent after a Polya operation as compared to a Billroth I. Anaemic patients who are iron deficient are also likely to have low Cbl levels and iron therapy often produces a rise in the Cbl level. Again megaloblastic patients after partial gastrectomy have higher Cbl levels than pernicious anaemia patients.

Surprisingly there is not a good correlation between those who have low Cbl levels and their ability to absorb Cbl. In fact, a quarter of patients after gastrectomy who have an impaired Cbl absorption test, have normal serum Cbl levels, and the absorption of Cbl is apparently normal in over 30% of those with low Cbl levels.

Clinically, iron deficiency may alter the presentation of megaloblastic anaemia after partial gastrectomy very significantly as indicated in Chapters 4 and 10. In more than half the patients iron therapy alone may restore a low Cbl level to within the normal range but a rise in the Cbl level is relatively slow over 10–20 weeks.

Cbl deficiency can produce severe symptoms in patients after partial gastrectomy who remain normoblastic with normal or marginally iron-deficient indices. A reduced Cbl level with evidence of malabsorption is an indication for Cbl therapy after partial gastrectomy.

Vagotomy and pyloroplasty

Although about 10% of patients may become iron deficient after vagotomy, particularly when combined with gastroenterostomy, serum Cbl levels and Cbl absorption remain normal. Megaloblastic anaemia has not been described.

Gastric surgery for obesity

Bypass of the stomach is brought about by creating a small gastric pouch at the oesophogeal end and the rest of the stomach is bypassed by a gastrojejunostomy. The procedure severely limits dietary intake because the amount of food taken is limited by the size of the pouch and its stoma. No increase in gastritis was found among 34 patients followed up for an average of 22 months [128] who had undergone a vertical banded gastroplasty.

However, 54 sera taken from 178 patients (30%) had low Cbl levels [129–131]. Malabsorption of Cbl (1.0 µg) was present in 8 of 15 patients [129]. Red cell folate was low in 3 of 17 patients [131].

One case of megaloblastic anaemia diagnosed 6 years after operation has been reported [132]. This patient had a low Cbl level, malabsorbed Cbl and the absorption of Cbl improved with added IF.

Chapter 12 Nutritional cobalamin deficiency

Cobalamin is entirely absent from the plant kingdom and hence a strictly vegetarian diet does not supply Cbl. Diets are almost never so restrictive as to avoid all sources of Cbl and even if food of obvious animal origin is excluded, microbial contamination of food or drinking water supplies some Cbl. Although there are isolated case reports of megaloblastic anaemia among strict, generally Caucasian, vegetarians, the bulk of the population at risk are the many millions of strict Hindus who for religious reasons are lifelong vegetarians. The emigration of large numbers of such Indian subjects to the UK from East Africa in the 1960s made it possible to study such patients in detail [16, 133–135].

A study of serum Cbl levels in relation to diet showed a mean Cbl level of 430 pg/ml among non-vegetarians, 320 pg/ml among 'semi' vegetarians, 230 pg/ml among lacto-ovo vegetarians, 190 pg/ml among lacto vegetarians and 120 pg/ml among total vegetarians (vegans) [137].

Among 1000 Hindu Indians living in London, the mean serum Cbl level was 198 pg/ml and 54% had a 'low' level, that is below 170 pg/ml [16].

Not only is there a high frequency of Cbl deficiency among Hindu vegetarians but also a high frequency of iron deficiency due to poor availability of iron from a vegetarian diet, a high frequency of osteomalacia due to low intake of calcium and vitamin D and a frequency of tuberculosis that is 38 times higher than in Caucasians [16]. The haematology is often complicated by co-existing alpha- or beta-thalassaemia trait as well as by iron deficiency.

Over a 14-year period 138 Gujerati Hindu patients with megaloblastic anaemia were seen at one hospital [16]. The diagnosis of dietary Cbl deficiency was made by either a haematological response to oral Cbl (generally 5 µg daily) or a response to parenteral Cbl in a patient who had normal Cbl absorption.

The commonest complaints on presentation were lethargy, dyspnoea on exertion, loss of appetite and loss of weight. Generalized pains due to osteomalacia were present in 19%. Paraesthesiae were present in 10% and a sore tongue and mouth in 7%. Some presented with infertility (5%) and some with unexpected macrocytosis in a blood count (6%). Of the 138 patients studied, 100 had nutritional Cbl deficiency and 20 Addisonian pernicious anaemia. Only four had primary folate deficiency which was nutritional in origin though complicated by alcoholism in two. The age at presentation of patients with nutritional Cbl deficiency ranged from 13 to 83 years and the severity of anaemia was equally wide with haemoglobin levels below 6 g/dl in 13 patients and above 14 g/dl in another 13. Although the majority had a raised MCV up to 130 fl, 15 did not due to an accompanying beta-thalassaemia trait in five, alpha-thalassaemia trait in two and accompanying iron deficiency in eight. All had a megaloblastic marrow which was the basis of diagnosis.

As in untreated pernicious anaemia, intestinal malfunction was present in one-third of patients as shown by increased faecal fat excretion (Fig. 2.9) and impaired xylose absorption. Impaired Cbl absorption was present in five patients with nutritional Cbl deficiency, and in three who were retested several months after Cbl therapy, normal Cbl absorption had been restored. All other patients with nutritional Cbl deficiency absorbed Cbl normally.

Treatment of nutritional Cbl deficiency in the long term is by persuading the patients to broaden their diets which is possible among younger educated Indians but impossible among older subjects who have a distaste for foods of animal origin apart from any religious objection. In these a daily oral Cbl supplement is recommended and one is marketed supplying 50 µg Cbl. Parenteral Cbl does not appear to be justified when the patient is able to absorb Cbl normally.

The high frequency of tuberculosis has been ascribed to the impaired killing of *M. tuberculosis* by macrophages that are both Cbl and iron deficient. Such deficiencies impair the oxygen burst that is the mechanism of intracellular killing [138].

There are various estimates of the Cbl content of a diet consumed by vegetarians. These range from 0.3 to 0.4 µg/day [139], 0.5 µg [133] and 0.8 µg [7]. All the patients with nutritional Cbl deficiency had low serum Cbl levels, 31 out of 78 had low red cell folate levels [16] although none required folate therapeutically. Eighty-seven out of the 138 patients with megaloblastic anaemia had clinically overt iron deficiency at some time and many required iron in addition to Cbl.

Cbl neuropathy was present in only one Indian patient with pernicious anaemia [16] and a possible example in a vegan of 25 years duration has been described [140].

Nutritional Cbl deficiency in infants of Cbl-deficient mothers

In India a disorder has been described in breast-fed infants with abnormal skin pigmentation, retarded development and megaloblastic anaemia. The mothers were vegetarian and the anaemia in the infant generally responded to Cbl [141, 142]. Cbl is normally transferred to the fetus *in utero* in the last few weeks of pregnancy when there is avid accumulation of Cbl in the placenta. Cord blood Cbl levels are significantly higher than maternal levels (240 and 373 pg/ml in mothers and cord blood) [435]. When the mother is deficient in Cbl because of a strict vegetarian diet or because of undetected pernicious anaemia, fetal Cbl stores are low. The Cbl level in breast milk is the same as that in maternal plasma. When the mothers serum Cbl level is low, that in breast milk is equally low and Cbl deficiency develops in the infant. Deficiency in the infant can be treated by giving Cbl to the infant or by giving Cbl to the mother where the Cbl level in breast milk will rise to an extent that a haematological response ensues in the infant [142].

There are at least six reports among Caucasian mothers who adhered to strict vegetarian diets and whose offspring presented with severe megaloblastic anaemia due to the failure of supply of Cbl from breast milk [144–149]. The mothers had been strict vegetarians for between 5 and 12 years and were all clinically well. The infants all developed normally for the first 4 months of life but thereafter declined and presented clinically between 6 and 12 months. The infants were lethargic but hyperirritable. They were weak, could not support their heads nor turn over. They stopped smiling, became inactive and withdrawn. One infant had evidence of neuropathy with marked muscle hypotonia, exaggerated reflexes, positive flexor plantar responses, partial optic atrophy, diffuse brain atrophy and was in coma on presentation [149]. Some remain of normal weight but most are underweight. Increased pigmentation on the backs of the hands and the feet most marked over the knuckles may occur [149]. One child was in congestive cardiac failure [147]. The haemoglobin level on presentation ranged from 2.2 to 7.3 g/dl in five infants and was 13.0 g/dl in the sixth. Most had a raised MCV, low serum Cbl levels and severely megaloblastic marrows. Methylmalonylaciduria and homocystinuria were present in one infant [145] but this was probably not looked for in the other cases. The response to parenteral Cbl was dramatic in all cases with marked clinical improvements within days and rapid restoration of normal blood values within a few weeks.

Although pernicious anaemia in the mother is usually associated with infertility, mild Cbl deficiency is still rarely compatible with an apparently normal pregnancy. As in vegetarian mothers, the infant has significantly reduced Cbl stores, fails to thrive and anaemia is found in the first few months of life. This was first described in 1954 [143] and there have been at least six other reports since [150–154]. Presentation was between 4 and 14 months of life essentially as described in infants of mothers with nutritional Cbl deficiency. The haemoglobin levels have ranged from 3.0 to 9.4 g/dl and several have had raised urinary levels of methylmalonic acid [152, 153]. The mothers were well clinically but in all haematological evidence of pernicious anaemia was present. One mother had attended an infertility clinic for 10 years before conceiving [151]. The response of the infants to parenteral Cbl was prompt and complete.

Chapter 13   Disease of the small gut

Anatomical abnormalities (blind loop syndrome)

The absence of a permanent bacterial flora in the stomach and small intestine is due to a combination of factors: the low pH of gastric juice, the secretion of immunoglobulin by lymphocytes in the gut wall, the secretion of bile acids, the motility of the gut which prevents stasis of contents and the effect of the ileocaecal valve in limiting reflux of colonic contents which have a profuse microflora. The normal upper gut contains less than 10 000 bacteria per ml except after meals when there is a transient increase. In poor hygienic conditions and in tropical countries a more abundant and diverse flora including coliforms are present in the small gut of apparently healthy persons. In such populations the small intestinal villi are shorter and wider than in subjects from temperate climates.

The factors that lead to bacterial contamination of the bowel are listed below.

Intestinal stasis

1 *Anatomical defects*: diverticuli, strictures, fistulae, surgical blind loops.
2 *Impaired motility*: scleroderma, Whipples disease, postvagotomy, ganglion-blocking drugs.
3 *Impaired defences*: achlorhydria, immune deficiency, cholangitis, monosaccharide malabsorption, long-term use of H_2-antagonists.

When these mechanisms break down what has been termed 'the contaminated small bowel syndrome' develops. There is then malabsorption of fat and Cbl in association with excessive numbers of bacteria particularly anaerobes in the small intestine. In time Cbl deficiency and megaloblastic anaemia develop.

Fat absorption

The steatorrhoea present in the blind loop syndrome may in part be related to poor miscelle formation attributed to bacterial deconjugation of bile acids but possibly also to mucosal damage demonstrated in the brush border of jejunal

101

biopsies. Low levels of enzymes normally produced by enterocytes have been demonstrated in both the experimental and clinical situation [155].

Cobalamin absorption

Impaired Cbl absorption is one of the most consistent findings in bowel bacterial overgrowth. The micro-organisms simply abstract Cbl from ingested food and hence it is unavailable to the host. Gram-negative anaerobes readily take up the Cbl–IF complex whereas aerobes such as *S. faecalis* largely take up free Cbl. But as Cbl dissociates from IF free Cbl will be available from the complex. In a few patients alteration of the Cbl molecule into inactive forms by bacteria was demonstrated [156]. Provided that the ileum remains intact, impaired Cbl absorption in the blind loop syndrome is reversed temporarily by antibiotics such as tetracycline or colistin.

Folate status

One of the remarkable features of the blind loop syndrome is that although the microflora have a stupendous appetite for Cbl they do not deprive the host of folate. In culture of these organisms, folate tends to acumulate in the medium and clinically such patients may have raised serum folate levels and increased folate excretion in urine. These raised serum folates fall after a course of appropriate antibiotic [157]. Intestinal absorption of folate is generally normal. In 12 patients undergoing gastric bypass surgery although the mean folate intake fell from 253 to 65 µg folate daily, the serum folate rose from 3.8 to 10.4 ng/ml [158].

The lesion

Clinically the gut lesion may be intestinal strictures (tuberculous, post-operative adhesions, regional enteritis, carcinoma, trauma or of unknown causation), anastomoses and fistulae (entero-entero, entero-colostomy or gastro-jejunocolic), small intestinal diverticulosis or stagnant loops (post-surgical, regional ileitis and tuberculosis).

Scleroderma impairs gut mobility. Hypogammaglobulinaemia results in lack of secretory IgA.

Clinical situation

Patients who develop a megaloblastic anaemia in association with an abnormal intestinal flora tend to have more prominent gastrointestinal symptoms than other patients with megaloblastic anaemia. These include dyspepsia, abdominal discomfort, distension, nausea and vomiting. There may be sub-acute intestinal obstruction and abdominal colic. In severe cases anorexia, weight loss and progressive weakness occurs. Borborygmi can be prominent and embarrassing. Diarrhoea may accompany steatorrhoea.

When Cbl deficiency supervenes glossitis and symptoms of anaemia appear. Particularly in small intestinal diverticulitis Cbl neuropathy may be present. Examination in addition to features of megaloblastic anaemia may show a distended abdomen with scars of previous surgery. Abdominal sounds and even visible peristalsis may be evident.

Megaloblastic anaemia in the blind loop syndrome was described almost 100 years ago. The age of patients ranges from 8 to 85 but it is unusual to see anaemia with small gut diverticulosis under the age of 50. Up to 10 years may elapse between a surgical procedure and megaloblastic anaemia [7].

Megaloblastic anaemia occurs in the majority of cases of established blind loop syndrome. Malabsorption of Cbl is the rule and anaemia is due to Cbl deficiency. Impaired Cbl absorption is not improved by repeating the test with added IF but is improved after a course of appropriate antibiotic.

Investigation requires demonstration of the lesion by radiology. Increased urinary indican is useful confirmatory evidence of intestinal bacterial overgrowth as is detection in the breath of $^{14}CO_2$ following ingestion of ^{14}C-labelled substrates metabolized by bacteria such as xylose or bile acids. Direct aerobic and anaerobic culture of small bowel contents collected under meticulous conditions provides a quantitative as well as qualitative assessment of flora [155].

Treatment of megaloblastic anaemia is with parenteral Cbl. Surgical reversal of any structural abnormality where possible, should be done. Intermittent antibiotics may be useful using tetracycline, metronidazole, lincomycin or cotrimoxazole. Neomycin is not effective. Particular cases require nutritional support [159].

Jejunoileal bypass   This operation enjoyed a vogue in the treatment of obesity. Proximal jejunum was anastomosed to the distal ileum bypassing the bulk of the small gut. An abnormal gut flora appeared in the upper gut and the serum Cbl level fell being abnormally low in 68% of patients 5 years after the operation [160]. Two-thirds had serum folate levels below 7 ng/ml after 5 years. Impaired Cbl absorption was present in all six patients in one study [161] and was transiently improved with tetracycline. In another study Cbl absorption was depressed in all 11 patients but was still within the normal range in four [162]. Megaloblastic anaemia has not been reported.

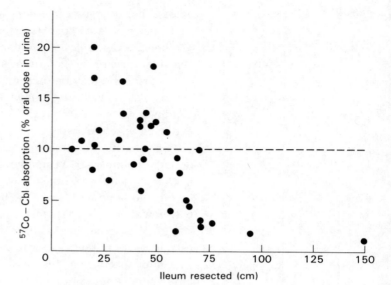

Fig. 13.1 Cbl absorption tests using the urinary excretion method carried out in patients who had undergone ileal resection shows that the more ileum that is removed the more likely is Cbl malabsorption to be present.

Ileal resection

Resection of significant amounts of ileum always interferes with the absorption of Cbl (Fig. 13.1). The amount of remaining ileum necessary to maintain Cbl absorption varies from patient to patient. One patient was able to absorb Cbl with only 38 cm of remaining ileum and generally absorption is normal if less than 60 cm is removed. The majority of patients who have more than 60 cm resected have Cbl malabsorption [163]. When in addition to removing ileum jejunum is removed, then steatorrhoea as well as Cbl malabsorption ensues. Folate absorption remains normal.

When Cbl replacement is not given, Cbl deficiency and megaloblastic anaemia develops and in 11 patients with extensive resection six had Cbl deficiency after 5 years with Cbl neuropathy in three [164].

Children appear to adapt to massive resection better than adults. Twelve children who had over 45 cm of ileum removed usually as neonates grew normally after the first year and nine had normal serum Cbl levels several years later [165], although six had impaired Cbl absorption.

Ileal irradiation

Loops of distal ileum are normally present in the pelvis and hence pelvic irradiation is very likely to produce radiation damage to these segments of bowel. Such irradiation may be given to treat carcinoma of the cervix uteri or the bladder. At laparotomy such irradiated bowel appears white, rigid and thickened. Histologically there is marked oedema of the gut wall with fibrosis. A high proportion of patients fail to absorb Cbl after pelvic irradiation. This was the case in eight out of 14 [166] and in five out of 13 patients [167] in two series. A low serum Cbl level was present in ten out of 41 patients treated for carcinoma of the bladder [167]. Serum folate levels were normal. In addition some patients develop steatorrhoea and diarrhoea [168, 169] although most are asymptomatic [166].

Megaloblastic anaemia was described in a 71-year-old woman who had undergone pelvic irradiation for carcinoma of the cervix 9 years previously [170]. The anaemia responded completely to parenteral Cbl. She failed to absorb either Cbl given alone, or with IF or after tetracycline. The damaged segment of ileum was biopsied when she underwent a laparotomy for carcinoma of the colon at the time that she developed megaloblastic anaemia. Pernicious anaemia was excluded by the presence of a normal gastric mucosa and the presence of acid and IF in the gastric secretion.

Regional enteritis (Crohn's disease)

The region of gut most frequently involved in Crohn's disease is the distal one-quarter of the small intestine and the proximal colon. In time more than half the patients require intestinal resection of varying extent. In the absence of gut resection it remains surprising how infrequent megaloblastic anaemia is in these patients and it is only in those patients who have undergone relatively large ileal resections that severe malabsorption of Cbl develops.

A macrocytic or megaloblastic anaemia was reported among 84 out of 392 patients (21%) [7]. There are two reports of Cbl neuropathy in patients who had both undergone resection and been given oral folate [171, 172]. The serum Cbl level was found to be low in 104 out of 542 patients (19%) in eight combined series [173]. Cbl absorption was abnormal, using the urinary excretion test, in 128 out of 281 patients (46%) in five series [7, 174, 175]. There did not appear to be a great correlation between the extent of disease and Cbl absorption but a good correlation with the length of ileum that had been resected. Thus among 47 patients who had had less than 30 cm ileum resected, only two apparently malabsorbed Cbl; abnormal results were found in 20 out of 44 patients (45%) who had 30–60 cm resected and in 17 out of 30 patients who had more than 90 cm resected [174]. Low serum Cbl levels tended to occur in those who had undergone resection.

Low serum folate levels have been reported in 207 out of

545 patients (38%) and low red cell folates in 41 out of 169 patients (24%) [173]. Factors that predispose to the development of folate deficiency include anorexia, malabsorption, active disease and effects of sulphasalazine used in treatment. Sulphasalazine may interfere with folate absorption as well as causing haemolysis. Folate deficiency has been noted as an invariable feature of diffuse jejuno-ileal disease [176].

Impaired folate absorption has been reported in Crohn's disease although results vary with the methods used [7].

Crohn's disease of the stomach is reported to have led to a Cbl-deficient megaloblastic anaemia analogous to that found in pernicious anaemia [177].

Infestation with the fish tapeworm

A number of parasitic helminths concentrate large amounts of Cbl in their anterior segments where it is converted into adenosylcobalamin. There it functions as a coenzyme in the isomerization of succinyl-CoA to methylmalonyl-CoA, a step required in the production of propionate. There does not appear to be any methylCbl in this species. Receptor sites for Cbl have been identified on the brush border of outer cell membranes along the entire length of the cat tape work [178].

Diphyllobothrium latum (fish tapeworm) is a parasite of man (and dog) and is acquired by eating fresh water fish harbouring larva of the tapeworm. Heating above 51–55°C will kill the larva as will freezing below −10°C. Thus infection occurs through eating raw or undercooked fish. Infestation was rife in Finland and the Baltic states although occasional cases are described from infected salmon in North America [179] and Chile [180]. Tapeworm ova appear in the faeces of the host 5–6 weeks after eating inadequately cooked fish.

In Finland, 40 years ago, 20% of the population harboured the tapeworm. Successful pollution of the fresh water lakes however appears to have reduced the numbers of fish considerably and with this there has been a decline in patients presenting with anaemia. Prior to this some 9% of carriers had megaloblastic marrows and a further 8% giant metamyelocytes. Cbl neuropathy was present among 8% of carriers. Just over one-third to half of the carriers had a serum Cbl level below 100 pg/ml [7].

Impaired Cbl absorption was present in 92% of tapeworm carriers although a later study found a lower frequency of 54% of Cbl malabsorption [7], a difference no doubt due to better urine collection in the second study.

In patients with megaloblastic anaemia, where the worm

was attached high up the small gut, between 83 and 100% of a dose of $[^{57}Co]B_{12}$ was recovered from the worm. When the worm was lodged lower down the gut generally in non-anaemic subjects, there was a smaller uptake of labelled Cbl by the worm — generally about 40% of an 0.5 µg dose. The amount of Cbl in the worm ranged from 1.3 to 3.0 µg/g. The worm could readily take up Cbl given bound to IF [181, 182].

Megaloblastic anaemia due to the fish tapeworm was described more than 100 years ago. Remission ensued following expulsion of the worm. The youngest affected patient was 9-years-old. The signs and symptoms are the same as those found in pernicious anaemia. A sub-optimal haematological response follows worm expulsion with niclosamide (0.5 g orally) with subjective improvement within 2 weeks. Both neuropathy and the blood responded. Rapid response requires both parenteral Cbl combined with worm expulsion. The serum Cbl levels rise slowly after worm expulsion alone and continue to rise for several years.

Coeliac disease (gluten-sensitive enteropathy)

This disorder is characterized by intestinal malabsorption and an abnormal jejunal mucosa which improves morphologically when gluten is withdrawn from the diet. Relapse follows re-introduction of gluten. It has a frequency of 1 in 2000 of the population but in some parts of Ireland the frequency reaches 1 in 300. Siblings may be affected in 10–20% of families.

Not less than half of untreated patients have anaemia. Iron deficiency predominates in children whereas folate deficiency predominates in adults. The anaemia is not due to Cbl deficiency, although there are rare exceptions [136], and cobalamin is virtually never required for a response. Some 20 years ago almost all patients had a megaloblastic anaemia but heightened awareness of the disease has led to diagnosis on criteria other than blood changes. A macrocytic blood picture is present in two-thirds of adult patients. The appearance of the blood film frequently reflects splenic atrophy that is a feature of coeliac disease and shows Howell–Jolly bodies and target cells. Some 10–20% of adults have an iron-deficiency anaemia on initial presentation. In the absence of other pointers to malabsorption, suspicion is raised by the absence of a cause for blood loss including hypomenorrhoea in women and a failure to respond to oral iron therapy. Among 122 coeliac patients 89% were anaemic and half had a haemoglobin concentration of less than 10 g/dl. Only three patients had simple iron deficiency and just under half had megaloblastic anaemia with some iron stores and just over half had megalo-blastosis combined with iron deficiency [183]. Most required iron for a complete response.

A low serum Cbl levels was present in 97 out of 231 (42%) untreated coeliac patients [7] and impaired Cbl absorption was present in 111 out of 272 (41%) patients. Cbl absorption is not influenced by the addition of IF, nor is it improved by antibiotic therapy. Generally those with a low Cbl level also have impaired Cbl absorption. However, the brunt of the disease is borne by the jejunum which makes first contact with dietary gluten and the ileum is usually affected far less severely. Thus Cbl deficiency rarely reaches clinical signi-ficance in coeliac disease. However, two examples of Cbl neuropathy have been noted, one patient having been treated with folic acid for 3 years [7, 184] and three other patients not only required Cbl therapy but Cbl malabsorption persisted on a gluten-free diet [136]. Coincidental pernicious anaemia may have been present.

In almost all patients with coeliac disease megaloblastic anaemia is due to folate deficiency and this, in turn, is due to folate malabsorption. Almost all patients have low serum folate levels [183] and almost all have low red cell folates [7]. Although the value of low red cell (and serum) folate in diagnosis has been questioned in children [7] the finding of normal folate status must place the diagnosis of coeliac disease very low in the list of probabilities. A persistently low serum folate in treated patients suggested non-compliance with a gluten-free diet [185]. Urinary formiminoglutamic acid excretion is almost invariably elevated.

Tests for folate absorption almost always give abnormal results in untreated coeliacs. Using [^{3}H]-labelled folate con-trols absorbed 85% of a 2 mg dose of folate whereas coeliacs only absorbed 29%. Impaired folate malabsorption affects both folate monoglutamate and folate polyglutamnate forms (Fig. 13.2). Following a gluten-free diet the absorption of both forms is restored [186]. Folate monoglutamates are better absorbed than polyglutamates in both controls and coeliac patients.

All the abnormalities found in coeliac patients are reversed albeit slowly by a successful gluten-free diet. Both folate and Cbl absorption become normal [7]. In practice improvement is hastened by oral folate and iron when required.

Dermatitis herpetiformis   This is a pruritic vesicular skin lesion treated with sulphones

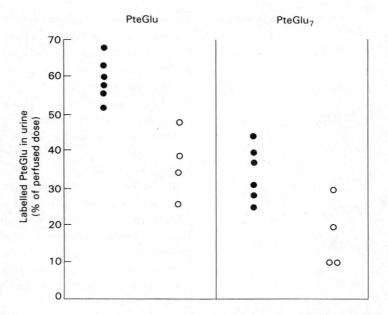

Fig. 13.2 Labelled folate was perfused through a jejunal segment in volunteers (●) and patients with coeliac disease (○). Thereafter a large injection of unlabelled folate was given which carried much of the absorbed labelled folate into urine. Folatemonoglutamate (PteGlu) was better absorbed than folatepolyglutamate (PteGlu$_7$) in both controls and coeliac patients. The absorption of folate in coeliac disease was impaired as compared to controls [186].

(dapsone). Patients have villus atrophy as in coeliac disease and this responds to a gluten-free diet. Anaemia tends to be haemolytic due to the direct toxic action of dapsone on red cells but in some patients can be megaloblastic due to folate deficiency. About three-quarters of patients have low serum folate levels and one-third low red cell folates [187]. Splenic atrophy may be present and about half the patients may malabsorb folate. Cbl status is unaffected [188].

Tropical malabsorption (sprue)

A form of intestinal malabsorption is rife in tropical areas other than tropical Africa. It frequently leads to megaloblastic anaemia due to either folate or Cbl deficiency and these haematinics with antibiotics remain the only effective forms of therapy. The causation remains poorly understood. The general view is that it is the end result of an abnormal gut flora producing damage to the enterocyte, the effects of which are aggravated by folate deficiency and undernutrition [189, 190]. Symptoms of chronic diarrhoea, malaise and weight loss accompany malabsorption of fat, carbohydrate, folate and Cbl in the fully developed case. Megaloblastic anaemia is present in between 60 and 90% of patients diagnosed as having tropical sprue [7] and the severity of the anaemia is largely related to the duration of the illness.

Caucasian expatriates

The earliest symptoms among 50 military personnel sent to the Far East was loss of appetite, often gross, leading to weight loss. Sore mouth and tongue developed in 40% as well as dyspepsia, flatulence and abdominal discomfort. Intense fatigue was prominent. Anaemia appeared after the illness had been present for 2–3 months and became quite severe in women. Marrows were megaloblastic in 80% of these patients. The longer the duration of the illness the lower the serum folate and serum Cbl levels (Fig. 13.3). Urinary formiminoglutamic acid was markedly elevated in those with a duration of illness longer than 3 months. Jejunal biopsies became increasingly abnormal with duration of illness. All had steatorrhoea and impaired xylose absorption. The majority had Cbl malabsorption as assessed by a faecal excretion technique.

A few patients underwent spontaneous remissions on hospitalization. Best responses were obtained to folic acid therapy. Occasionally a slow response was obtained to antibiotic therapy [191].

Overland travellers to India

Diarrhoea, abdominal distension and weight loss were presenting features in Caucasians making their way by land to

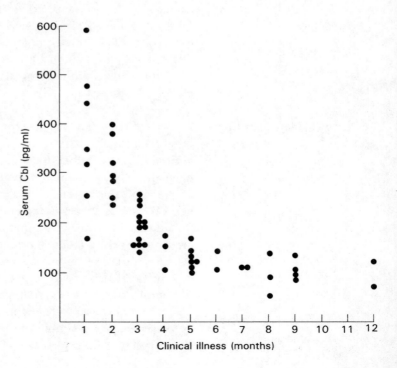

Fig. 13.3 The serum Cbl level declined with the duration of the clinical illness in soldiers who acquired tropical sprue.

India and eating local foods on route. The features were similar to those described among army personnel with malabsorption of fat, xylose and Cbl the rule. There was a response to tetracycline most evident after 4 weeks [192].

Endemic sprue in southern India

This presents at all ages with diarrhoea, anorexia and abdominal discomfort or pain. Although the diarrhoea might decline, patients continue to have malabsorption. Night blindness, sore tongue, hyperpigmentation and weight loss appear in those with illness of longer duration. Fifty-nine per cent had Cbl malabsorption but only 13% had folate malabsorption. Eighty per cent of patients were anaemic and 64% of marrows were megaloblastic.

A low serum Cbl level was present in 45% of patients and a serum folate below 6 ng/ml was present in 71% of patients. General measures including rehydration as well as folate, Cbl and antibiotics generally produced slow responses [193].

Endemic sprue in Puerto Rico

Clinical presentation is the same as described above. There is considerable variation in the severity of illness from mild when it is difficult to diagnose to very severe. An abnormal jejunal biopsy, steatorrhoea and abnormal radiological appearance in a barium series were present in well over 90% of patients and abnormal xylose and vitamin A absorption in over 80%. Megaloblastic marrow changes were present in even mild disease of short duration and disappeared on folate therapy. Cbl deficiency was not a factor in early disease [194]. Large doses of oral folate (15 mg/day) or Cbl in disease of longer duration produced rapid improvement. However, malabsorption of Cbl persisted despite improvement in other parameters even for years.

Other areas

Similar syndromes have been described in Haiti, Zambia, Natal in South Africa, West India, Pakistan and Vietnam.

Chapter 14 Inherited disorders of cobalamin and folate metabolism and disorders presenting in early life

The appearance of a small child with severe anaemia that reveals itself to be megaloblastic is usually unexpected. Some pre-planning is required to ensure that the correct samples are collected so that there is a minimum of delay before therapy is given. The disorders that present with megaloblastic anaemia in early life are as follows.

1 Usually presenting in the first 4 months.
    Transcobalamin II deficiency.
    Folate malabsorption.
    Inborn errors of cobalamin utilization.
    Thiamine-responsive megaloblastic anaemia.
    Orotic aciduria.
    Folate deficiency in premature infants.
2 Usually presenting in the first year.
    Intrinsic factor deficiency.
    Non-functional intrinsic factor.
    Cbl malabsorption (Imerslund–Gräsbeck).
    Maternal deficiency of cobalamin (Chapter 12).
    Goat's milk anaemia.
3 Presenting in the first decade or later.
    Pernicious anaemia (Chapter 10).
    Nutritional Cbl deficiency (Chapter 12).
    Coeliac disease (Chapter 13).
    Anticonvulsant drugs (Chapter 19).
    Purine nucleoside phosphorylase deficiency.
    Lesch–Nyhan syndrome.
    Impaired folate uptake.

In addition there are disorders of Cbl and folate metabolism that do not cause a megaloblastic anaemia but may be associated with impaired mental development or even neuropathy. These include the following.
    R-binder deficiency.
    Formimino-transferase deficiency.
    Methylenetetrahydrofolate reductase deficiency.

Methylmalonylaciduria.

Sarcosinaemia.

In severe megaloblastic anaemia in small children there is strong pressure to initiate treatment. If it is not possible to delay treatment even for 24 hours then blood should be collected for serum transcobalamin II (TCII), serum Cbl and serum folate levels, red cell folate as well as for a full blood count and a biochemical screen. Urine is examined particularly for proteinuria.

A marrow sample is taken to determine morphology and, if possible, to carry out a dU suppression test. Then 5 mg folic acid and 250 µg OHCbl are given by injection.

If it is possible to delay treatment for 24 hours then a 24-hour urine collection is made for methylmalonic acid, homocysteine and orotic acid. In any event even if treatment has to be given the urine in the first 24 hours is still collected for these parameters. Where treatment can be delayed it may also be useful to delay the marrow in order that arrangements can be made for the performance of a dU suppression test since this test may not be available on site.

Thereafter treatment is continued until it becomes evident which deficiency is present. Blood samples should also be collected from both parents for a full blood count, TCII and Cbl levels. In time it may be necessary to do absorption tests with labelled Cbl and with folate and to examine gastric juice. A fibroblast culture may be needed for study of Cbl utilization and it's coenzyme activity.

Transcobalamin II deficiency

TCII is the principal Cbl transport protein. It transports Cbl out of the enterocyte to portal blood and is required for uptake of Cbl by liver, marrow and other cells of the body. Only about 10% of TCII in plasma carries Cbl. The bulk (90%) of plasma Cbl is on R-binder. Total absence of functional TCII results in a failure of Cbl absorption and the absence of Cbl from cells results in severe megaloblastic anaemia.

About 20 cases of megaloblastic anaemia due to TCII have been investigated. The classical presentation is of an infant between 6 weeks to 3 months of age who fails to thrive and loses weight. Diarrhoea and vomiting is frequent. Examination shows a pale apathetic infant. The tongue may be red. There may be mouth ulcers. Anaemia may be very severe with a grossly megaloblastic marrow, leucopenia and thrombocytopenia. The serum Cbl level remarkably is normal or even raised. Serum folate may be raised. The reason for the

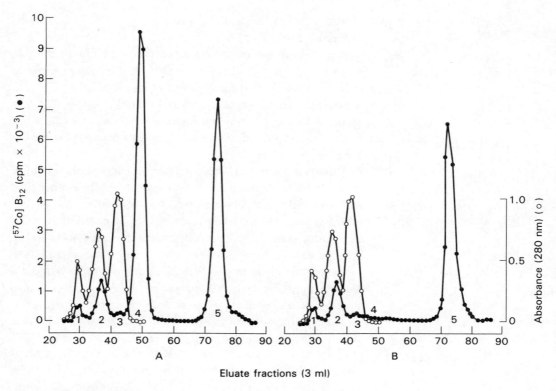

Fig. 14.1 ^{57}Co–B$_{12}$ is added to serum and this is eluted through a Sephacryl S-200 gel filtration column. The eluate fractions are collected, their absorbance at 280 nm read and the ^{57}Co–B$_{12}$ content counted. The protein (○) and ^{57}Co–B$_{12}$ (●) are plotted. 1, TC 0; 2, R-binder; 3, albumin; 4, TCII; 5, free ^{57}Co–B$_{12}$. A is a result from normal serum; B shows the total absence of a TCII peak seen in TCII deficiency.

normal concentration of serum Cbl is that it is carried on R-binder and TCII is required to take Cbl off the binder before it can be used. In the absence of TCII the Cbl on R-binder is unavailable.

Most cases do not have increased amounts of methyl-malonic acid in the urine but a few do. A few children have evidence of neuropathy [195] and failure of proper treatment in some has led to impaired mental development. There may be a history of a similarly affected sibling.

Since TCII in plasma is responsible for most of the Cbl uptake when Cbl is added to plasma, the plasma unsaturated Cbl-binding capacity is very low indeed. Column chromatography reveals the absence of a protein peak binding labelled Cbl in the position normally occupied by TCII (Fig. 14.1). But increasingly when immunological methods are used to measure TCII detectable TCII is present which presumably is non-functional [196–199]. Much has been made in the literature of immunological defects but these disappear on Cbl treatment and any persistence simply reflects chronic undertreatment.

Parents have half the normal level of TCII and inheritance is that of an autosomal recessive trait. Polyacrylamide gel electrophoresis of TCII reveals a number of isoproteins. The technique depends on Cbl binding by these isoproteins followed by autoradiography. Since TCII-deficient patients do not bind Cbl this procedure cannot be carried out. However, investigation of parents showed that both isoprotein bands present in heterozygotes were equally depressed [200].

Response to treatment with Cbl is rapid and dramatic but relapse too is rapid when treatment is discontinued. High plasma Cbl levels following large doses of parenteral Cbl allows Cbl to enter cells by passive diffusion. Such high Cbl levels can be achieved only by frequent parenteral doses of Cbl, for example 1000 μg OHCbl twice weekly. Oral therapy does not deliver high doses to plasma (only 1% is absorbed) and less frequent injections produces the distressing blood picture of plunging and rising leucocytes, platelets and haemoglobin levels as haemopoiesis alternates between a normoblastic and megaloblastic state [201]. Such patients in the end are likely to become mentally impaired. Neuropathy has developed in a child maintained on oral therapy.

A number of interesting variants of TCII deficiency have been described usually in older and even adult patients. Cases have presented at 2, 4, 12, 32 and 39 years of age [196, 202, 203] and these patients have been able to absorb Cbl normally. Their TCII clearly had activity *in vivo* not only in the transport of Cbl from the gut but also in facilitating cellular uptake of Cbl, hence the later clinical presentation. Nevertheless, *in vitro* their TCII did not bind labelled Cbl. In one patient TCII was present in fibroblast culture at about 25% of the level in control cells although none was detectable in serum [198].

Two patients had low serum Cbl levels. One was diagnosed at the age of 3 months but the other at 39 years of age. One of these had unusual R-binder complexes [204] and the other low total R-binder levels [202].

Another atypical presentation was of a 2½-month-old infant whose marrow showed very large myeloid precursors in the absence of erythroid precursors. Pancytopenia was present and the MCV remained normal. Cbl was given because of a deteriorating situation and was followed by an unexpected but dramatic response [205].

It is clear that these disorders involve a variety of abnormalities of TCII from almost totally non-functional (? absent)

TCII to partially functional TCII. Abnormalities of the receptor for TCII have been suggested [202].

Clinically a not uncommon situation is that treatment has to be initiated and a decisive diagnosis is not reached on the basis of material available for assay. Arrangements are made for sera to be assayed elsewhere. Misleading results will be obtained unless the Cbl injections have been stopped for possibly several weeks to ensure excretion of free Cbl and to allow apoCbl binders to accumulate. The measurement requires the detection of Cbl binders by the addition of label-led Cbl. If such binding sites are occupied by Cbl given as treatment, no labelled Cbl can bind. Thus TCII appears to be absent. The clue may be given by the simultaneous absence of a labelled R-binder peak. In healthy subjects TCII and R-binders are secreted continuously and apo-binders appear in plasma within minutes of disappearance of free Cbl from plasma following its excretion by the kidney. The situation in patients with TCII deficiency has not been investigated. A further check that parenteral therapy has been stopped a sufficient length of time to allow all free Cbl to disappear is to assay the serum Cbl level in the plasma. Finally column chromatography is required and short cuts using QuSO, etc. are not recommended.

Abnormalities of R-type cobalamin binders

These glycoproteins (MW 56 000 to 62 000 daltons) are present in all body fluids. In plasma they carry the bulk of the endo-genous Cbl. Five examples of an absence of R-binder have been reported, all in adults [29]. These patients also lack R-binder in saliva and leucocytes. There is no disturbance of haemopoiesis. Most have come to notice because of an un-explained low serum Cbl level, and by screening patients with low Cbl level a further five examples were found [29]. Two of these five patients had neurological abnormalities and a third had multiple sclerosis. Another patient with absent R-binders had neurological abnormalities considered by the authors to be compatible with Cbl neuropathy [29]. A fourth patient, an alcoholic, had peripheral neuropathy and epi-lepsy. Atypical multiple sclerosis was said to be present in the first example of R-binder deficiency reported in 1969 [206]. It has thus been suggested that R-binder deficiency may be the basis of a neuropathy. R-binders can bind to a wide variety of Cbl analogues *in vitro*. A hypothetical role for R-binders as a mechanism for protecting man against potentially harmful Cbl analogues and the breakdown of such a mechanism as the means by which neuropathy arises, has been proposed [29]. However, deleterious effect of Cbl analogues in man or mammals has not been demonstrated.

Folate malabsorption

Some eight examples of congenital failure to absorb folate have been recorded all but one in girls. All presented with severe megaloblastic anaemia in the first few months of life, the oldest being 5 months. Parents are often consanguineous and other children may have died at an early age. The megaloblastic anaemia is due to folate deficiency and requires parenteral folate therapy. Clinically they are similar to children with TCII deficiency or other severe megaloblastic anaemia occurring at this age.

In addition to impaired transport of all folate analogues into the enterocyte there is a failure to transport methylfolate into the brain. There is progressive deterioration of the CNS, profound mental retardation, calcification of basal ganglia and epilepsy [207–209] However this is not always so and somes cases have been only mildly mentally impaired [210] or mentally normal [211]. In addition the last patient had a history of recurrent infections of the respiratory tract, lungs, ear and GI tract. There was evidence of deficiency of both cellular and humoral immunity.

Folate levels in CSF are very low varying from 0 to 2.8 ng/ml [208, 212].

The test that is done to establish the diagnosis is to measure

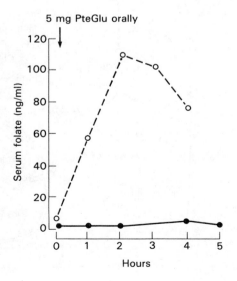

Fig. 14.2 An oral dose of 5 mg pteroylglutamic acid is given and blood samples collected before and at hourly intervals after the dose. A normal child shows a considerable rise in plasma folate (dashed line) assayed microbiologically. A child with congenital folate malabsorption barely shows a rise from baseline (solid line).

the change in plasma folate over a 2-hour period or longer following an oral dose of 5 mg folic acid. Normally this exceeds 100 ng/ml plasma at 1 or 2 hours. In these patients there is barely a rise (Fig. 14.2).

It has been suggested that parenteral folinic acid is advantageous in treatment [212]. Methylfolate would be even better since this is the analogue transported by the choroid plexus into CSF. Whatever the analogue relatively large doses (10–15 mg) should be given at least twice a week in the early years of life and thereafter cautious studies on whether a less frequent dose might suffice, be done. Plasma folate levels between injections might be a guide.

The underlying defect is not known but it is possibly due to an impaired folate receptor or transport protein.

Methylmalonylaciduria and homocystinuria — disorders of Cbl utilization

These disorders present either as a severe megaloblastic anaemia in early life usually with methylmalonylaciduria and homocystinuria, or with methylmalonylaciduria and homocystinuria in the absence of anaemia or with less severe megaloblastosis, or with only homocystinuria and megaloblastic anaemia. Diagnosis can be made from fibroblast cultures derived from the patient and prenatal diagnosis can be made from culture of amniocytes and even pre-natal cobalamin

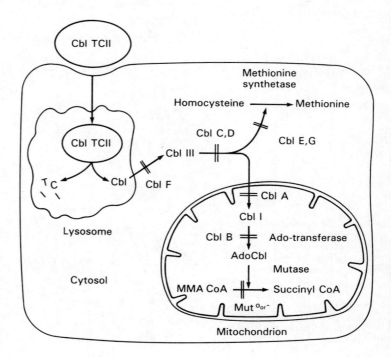

Fig. 14.3 A cell illustrating the site of the biochemical defect in disorders of Cbl metabolism producing methylmalonylaciduria and/or homocysteinuria. The defects (Cbl mutants A to G) are shown as double lines (see text).

therapy has been used [213, 214]. Those with only methyl-malonylaciduria include Cbl A,B and F mutants as well as defects in the enzyme methylmalonly-CoA mutase; those with methylmalonylaciduria and homocystinuria include Cbl C and D mutants, and Cbl E and G mutants show only homo-cystinuria. The disorders are better understood by relating them to the proposed underlying lesions (Fig. 14.3) which are as follows.

1 Lysosomal trapping of Cbl (Cbl F).
2 Impaired synthesis of adenosylCbl (Cbl A and B).
3 Impaired synthesis of methylCbl (Cbl E and G).
4 Impaired reduction of Cbl (Cbl C and D).
5 Abnormal methylmalonyl CoA-mutase.

The great majority of patients present in the first few months of life but some may present for the first time with mental deterioration in the second decade of life [215, 216]. Others with a defective mutase enzyme were discovered only by screening urine for methylmalonic acid in the absence of any clinical involvement [217].

Cbl A and B mutants (impaired AdoCbl formation)

The symptoms and signs in Cbl A and B mutants are the result of accumulation of methylmalonic acid. Accumulation of methylmalonic acid leads to acidosis and ketosis. The child fails to thrive, is lethargic, vomits and becomes dehydrated. There are difficulties in breathing, flaccidity of limbs and mental retardation. Severe cases may be in coma. There is hepatomegaly. There is increased ketones in blood and urine in 80% of patients, increased blood ammonia in 65% and anaemia, low platelets and low white cell count in up to half the patients. Ketoacidosis requires hydration with intra-venous glucose and bicarbonate.

A high proportion of these patients respond to Cbl therapy [216]. Ten out of 11 patients with the Cbl A mutant and three out of eight with the Cbl B mutant have responded with a marked fall in output of methylmalonic acid. However, al-though most of the Cbl A mutant patients are well, about a quarter are mentally impaired. Seventy per cent of Cbl A patients were alive and well 1–14 years after diagnosis. About 40% of Cbl B patients have died and an equal number do well [218].

The defect in Cbl A and Cbl B mutants is absence of active deoxyadenosyl Cbl. The explanation for this is not known in the case of Cbl A mutant but it has been suggested that there is impairment of the reductase converting Cob(III)alamin to

Cob(II)alamin and to Cob(I)alamin. Reduced cobalamin, however, is not required for the normal function of the mutase enzyme (it is not susceptible to oxidation by nitrous oxide) although adenosylation may require fully reduced cobalamin. In the case of Cbl B mutant there is impairment of Cob(I) alamin: ATP-adenosyltransferase so that synthesis of deoxyadenosylCbl is defective [219].

Cobalamin C and D mutants (impaired AdoCbl and methylCbl formation)

In these mutants accumulation of methylmalonic acid may cause ketoacidosis, accumulation of homocysteine may lead to thrombosis and there may be megaloblastic anaemia of varying severity. Neurological and psychiatric disorders may be prominent. Some 14 cases of Cbl C mutant have been described and one sibship with Cbl D mutant [220] has been described, one of the two brothers being clinically unaffected.

In those presenting in the first few weeks of life, lethargy and delayed mental development was present. Four patients out of 11 had microcephaly and two had seizures. Older patients presented with psychosis, delirium, spasticity and cerebral atrophy and three cases had perimacular retinal pigmentation which responded to Cbl. Some patients with Cbl C mutant have less dramatic symptoms and diagnosis has been suspected by screening of urine for methylmalonic acid. One neonate had multiple thromboses.

Marrows were noted to be megaloblastic in six cases and normoblastic in four. Serum Cbl and folate levels tend to be high. Cbl levels ranged from 285 to 2523 pg/ml and serum folate from 5.1 to 60 ng/ml. Most patients are moderately anaemic.

Most Cbl C mutant patients improved with injections of OHCbl (1 mg once or twice weekly) with decline in excretion of homocysteine and methylmalonic acid. Megaloblastic changes have usually regressed. Folinic acid was not useful but betaine (250 mg/kg/day) acted synergistically with OHCbl [221].

In Cbl C and D mutants cobalamin is not processed normally into the active coenzyme form. Both CH_3Cbl and AdoCbl are affected. It is assumed that the defect lies with the Cbl reductases. Cbl D differs from Cbl C mutant in that CNCbl could be converted to OHCbl in mixed fibroblast cultures (complementation) in the Cbl D mutant.

Cbl E and G mutants (impaired methylCbl formation)

These patients have homocystinuria only, the result of defects in the biosynthesis of methionine. These patients have megaloblastic anaemia. Four cases have been investigated.

Presentation is in the first few months of life with megaloblastic anaemia, homocysteine in urine and low plasma methionine levels [222]. The treatment is with large doses of OHCbl (1 mg daily to weekly). The Cbl G mutant is similar to Cbl E clinically. In both mutants there is impaired conversion of Cbl to CH_3Cbl, impaired incorporation of 5-methyltetrahydrofolate by fibroblasts and decreased methionine synthetase activity. The precise defect is not known. Cbl G and Cbl E are differentiated by complementation studies of fused fibroblasts. The defect in methionine synthesis is corrected when Cbl G cells are grown with Cbl E cells, indicating a different defect. The most recent example of Cbl G mutation was in a 21-year-old woman presenting with what appeared to be subacute combined degeneration of the cord with megaloblastic anaemia and a normal serum Cbl, serum folate and red cell folate levels [223].

Cbl F mutant (impaired Cbl release in lysosomes)

This patient developed stomatitis, glossitis, convulsions and hypotonia at 12 days of age. She was found to excrete excess methylmalonic acid in the urine but remained haematologically normal. Her fibroblasts accumulated Cbl in the lysosomes and failed to release it into the cytoplasm of the cell. In chloroquine-treated cells the Cbl remained in the lysosomes as a TCII–Cbl complex. The same phenomenon was observed in her cultured lymphocytes [224].

Her serum folate level was 49 ng/ml (raised). Although treated with OHCbl the child at 18 months was mentally retarded. She also has dextrocardia and dental abnormalities.

Investigation of cobalamin mutants

In addition to routine haematology and marrow morphology, Cbl and folate assays, dU suppression tests, measurement of transcobalamin and testing of urine for methylmalonic acid, homocysteine and orotic acid, further tests require setting up of fibroblast cultures. These can then be sent on to a laboratory equipped to carry out the appropriate studies (Table 14.1). These tests involve the following.

1 Incubation of [^{14}C]methyltetrahydrofolate with fibroblasts in the presence and absence of added OHCbl. The label in protein is assessed. This requires the transfer of the labelled methyl to methionine and the incorporation of methionine into cell protein. MethylCbl is the coenzyme of methionine synthetase.

2 Similarly incubation of fibroblasts with [^{14}C]propionate tests the methylmalonate pathway. Methylmalonate is converted to succinate, deoxyadenosylCbl being the coenzyme.

Table 14.1 Biochemical and clinical findings in inborn errors of cobalamin metabolism

Mutant	CblA	CblB	CblC	CblD	CblE	CblF	CblG
Clinical finding							
Megaloblastic anaemia	−	−	+	+	+	−	+
Mental retardation	−	−	±	+	+	±	±
Methylmalonylaciduria	+	+	+	+	−	+	−
Homocystinuria	−	−	+	+	+	±	+
Fibroblast studies							
[^{14}C]H$_3$H$_4$PteGlu fixation	+	+	−	−	−	?	
CH$_3$Cbl synthesis	+	+	−	−	−	±	−
AdoCbl synthesis	−	−	−	−	+	±	+
Conversion of CNCbl to OHCbl	+	+	−	±	−	−	
Lysosome transfer of Cbl	+	+	+	+	+	−	
Tissue extracts							
MMCoA mutase — holo	−	−	−	−	+	?	+
MMCoA mutase — total	+	+	+	+	+	?	+
Methionine synthetase holo	+	+	−	−	−	?	−
Methionine synthetase total	+	+	±	±	+	?	−
Cbl–adenosyl transferase	+	−	+	+	+	?	+

Succinate enters the Krebs cycle and its appearance in protein is monitored.

3 The concentration of AdoCbl and CH$_3$Cbl in fibroblasts after incubation with [^{57}Co]CNCbl is measured and compared with values in normal cells.

4 Extracts of the fibroblasts are used to measure methionine synthetase both in the absence of added CH$_3$Cbl (holoenzyme) and after CH$_3$Cbl addition (total enzyme).

5 Finally, mixed fibroblast cultures are set up in the presence of polyethylene glycol which promotes cell fusion. In this way failure of Cbl E fibroblasts to correct a biochemical defect found in the cell culture under investigation suggests that both cultures share the same defect. If correction occurs the defects are different.

Impaired methylmalonylCoA mutase

In addition to defects in the synthesis of adenosylCbl (Cbl A, Cbl B, Cbl C and Cbl D mutants) methylmalonylaciduria can arise from defects in the mutase apoenzyme. Their clinical presentation is similar to that described in relation to the Cbl A and Cbl B mutants. Biochemically in addition to methylmalonic acid in urine they have acidosis and ketosis, and raised levels of ammonia and of glycine [218]. They are normoblastic but the most severely affected patients have anaemia, leucopenia and less often thrombocytopenia. Patients with complete deficiencies of mutase apoenzyme (mut^0) presented earlier in infancy than other groups, indeed generally in the first week of life. Where there is some residual mutase activities (mut⁻) presentation was before 18 months [218].

With one doubtful exception none of the patients benefited from Cbl therapy [218] and most mut^0 patients die within 2 months. Thirty per cent of mut⁻ patients do better although an equal number have died.

Orotic aciduria This is a rare defect in pyrimidine synthesis transmitted as an autosomal recessive trait. Heterozygotes have partial deficiencies of the enzymes. Although only 11 cases have been described excellent responses to oral uridine occur and hence accurate diagnosis is important.

Children are found to have a severe megaloblastic anaemia, leucopenia, retarded growth and development and increased excretion in the urine of orotic acid. Most cases presented between 3 and 13 months of age but two were diagnosed at 3 and 7 years respectively. Indeed the 7-year-old patient showed normal growth and development [225–228]. Cbl and folate levels in blood are normal.

The pathway of pyrimidine synthesis involves the steps shown in Fig. 14.4.

In all but one of the patients enzymes marked 1 and 2 (orotate phosphoribosyltransferase and orotidine 5'phosphate decarboxylase respectively) have been reduced in activity. In one patient only orotidine 5'phosphate decarboxylase was impaired [228]. The loss of two adjacent enzymes suggests defect in the genetic control mechanism. Patients excrete 0.5–1.5 g orotic acid daily and crystals of orotic acid may appear in the urine deposit. Smaller increases in orotic acid may be seen in children with ornithine transcarboxylase deficiency with hyperammonaemia, in purine nucleoside phosphorylase deficiency and in lysine intolerance. In these orotic acid was absent in the fasting state but occurred after a

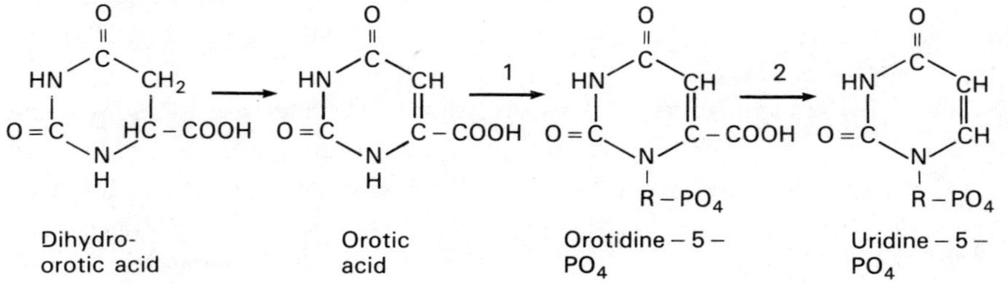

Fig. 14.4 In hereditary orotic aciduria there is impaired activity of enzymes orotate phosphoribosyltransferase (1) and orotidine-5'-phosphate decarboxylase (2).

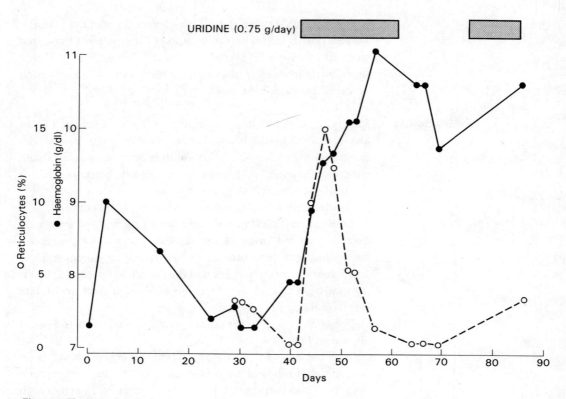

Fig. 14.5 The haematological response to uridine in hereditary orotic aciduria and relapse on its withdrawal.

protein load [229]. Orotic aciduria may also follow drugs such as 6-azauridine and allopurinol.

Heterozygotes were identified in 18 out of 63 members of one family [230]. The activities of the relevant enzymes were decreased in erythrocytes, leucocytes and fibroblast culture.

Oral uridine (1–1.5 g daily), which bypasses the enzyme block, restored normoblastic haemopoiesis (Fig. 14.5) and normal growth. After 2 years of uridine treatment erythrocyte phosphoribosyltransferase was reduced to 10% and after 3 years to 2% of normal activity [227, 228].

Lesch–Nyhan syndrome

This disorder is characterized by mental retardation, choreoathetosis and self-mutilation. There is impairment of synthesis of purine analogues other than adenine due to a lack of hypoxanthine phosphoribosyltransferase. A proportion of patients are macrocytic and megaloblastic and megaloblastosis has been seen in the mother of a patient. Haematological responses occur to adenine (1.5 g/day) with a reticulocytosis, a fall in the MCV and restoration of a normoblastic marrow but there is little clinical benefit from adenine therapy [231].

Relapse occurs on withdrawal of adenine. Low serum folate levels have been reported and ascribed to a high folate requirement due to markedly increased purine synthesis but these patients do not respond to folate.

Purine nucleoside phosphorylase deficiency

This enzyme deficiency may be associated with impaired function of T-lymphocytes. In two families the patients (15 months and 3 years) had megaloblastic marrows [232, 233] complicated in one by severe autoimmune haemolytic anaemia. Severe neuropathy may be present. Orotic acid in increased amounts may be present in urine. The child without haemolysis had a normal haemoglobin level.

Congenital intrinsic-factor deficiency

Over 50 examples of this disorder have been described [7, 234]. It usually presents in the first 2 years of life, occasionally in older patients, as a severe megaloblastic anaemia. These children deteriorate steadily after the first year of life with irritability, vomiting, diarrhoea and/or constipation, anorexia and listlessness leading to semi-coma.

The severely affected child is waxy and lemon-yellow in colour and well below its expected weight. There may be severe stomatitis with a smooth glazed tongue. Spleen and liver may be enlarged. Neuropathy may be present especially if folic acid has been prescribed. There may be loss of reflexes and vibration sense. Others are ataxic with brisk reflexes and extensor plantars. In the past these children had a series of relapses and remissions in the absence of clear diagnosis and systematic therapy. The parents may be related and several siblings may be affected.

Megaloblastic anaemia is present and blood is like that in untreated pernicious anaemia. The serum Cbl level is low. Cbl absorption tests give the same results as in pernicious anaemia.

These children differ from those with pernicious anaemia in that gastric mucosa is normal histologically, HCl and pepsin are present but IF is either absent or present in very low amounts. Their sera do not contain parietal-cell nor IF-antibodies and their parents and relatives do not show the high frequency of tissue antibodies present in pernicious anaemia relatives.

It is inherited as an autosomal recessive characteristic. They show dramatic responses to Cbl therapy and are treated in the long term in the same way as patients with pernicious anaemia.

Immunological methods demonstrated that proteins reacting with IF-antibodies were present in gastric biopsy specimens from six of nine patients. Thus there may be an inadequate synthesis of IF, a block to its secretion or secretion of an abnormal IF that either does not bind Cbl or, if it binds Cbl, does not promote its absorption [235]. No significant abnormality is present in the parents and parents who both have Addisonian pernicious anaemia do not produce offspring with congenital absence of IF.

An abnormal form of IF was present in a 13-year-old boy of a first cousin marriage. He presented with severe megaloblastic anaemia and had an IF-like protein in his gastric juice that bound labelled Cbl and reacted with IF-antibody. The IF failed to promote Cbl absorption both in the patient and in a volunteer who had undergone a total gastrectomy. An antiserum against the boy's gastric juice reacted with his parents' gastric juice, suggesting they were heterozygotes for an abnormal IF [236].

Another example of an abnormal IF was present in three siblings presenting with megaloblastic anaemia in their second decade of life. Their IF was abnormally sensitive to proteolysis in acid gastric juice [237].

Congenital cobalamin malabsorption (Imerslund–Gräsbeck)

This is by far the commonest form of megaloblastic anaemia occurring in early life and several hundred patients have been investigated. It is transmitted as an autosomal recessive trait and is not uncommon among inbred communities such as Lapps in Scandinavia and North African Jews. It is associated with proteinuria in 90% of patients. Although most cases present in the second year of life, in others diagnosis is made early in the second decade [7]. Clinical presentation is the same as described in relation to children with absent IF.

The blood and marrow is that of a classical megaloblastic anaemia, the serum Cbl level is low and the patient shows a full response to Cbl therapy. The gastric mucosa and gastric secretion are normal but there is impaired absorption of Cbl given alone, given with IF and given after antibiotics. The lesion appears to be in relation to the ileal Cbl–IF receptor. Ileal biopsy taken through a colonoscope showed failure of uptake of the Cbl–IF complex [238]. The jejunum and ileum are normal histologically. There is no other evidence of malabsorption.

The other interesting feature in this disorder is proteinuria. Renal biopsy and electron microscopy of the glomeruli showed considerable dilatation of the rough endoplasmic reticulum in the podocytes. Glomerular podocytes produce most of the capillary basement membrane material. It was thus suggested that the abnormality in the podocytes leads to a functionally abnormal basement membrane and hence an increase in permeability and proteinuria [239]. The link between an impaired ileal receptor for Cbl–IF and abnormal glomerular rough endoplasmic reticulum may be a defect in a pleiotropic gene or in two closely associated genes.

Treatment with Cbl, as in pernicious anaemia, is continued for life.

Goat's milk anaemia

Goat's milk has a relatively low content of both Cbl and folate; folate content is 6 µg/l (human 52 µg/l) and Cbl content is 0.1 µg/l (human 4 µg/l). Kids will eat grass within days of birth and are not dependent on maternal sources of supply. Human infants started on only goat's milk within a few weeks of birth get a severe megaloblastic anaemia at about 3–5 months due to folic acid deficiency [240]. Such cases were noted some 70 years ago and they continue to be reported. If goat's milk has to be used a folate supplement has to be added.

Thiamine-responsive megaloblastic anaemia

Some eight patients with thiamine-responsive megaloblastic anaemia, sensorineural deafness and diabetes mellitus have been described [241–245].

Deafness and diabetes requiring insulin preceded the finding of megaloblastic anaemia by several years. There was an equal sex distribution among the eight patients and in most the parents were cousins. Megaloblastic anaemia was noted before 3 months of age in two children but the others presented between 9 and 13 years. Haemoglobin levels varied from 6 to 10.3 g/dl and serum Cbl levels were normal. Serum folates were normal but one child had a low red cell folate level [244]. One child had congenital heart disease and another situs inversus.

In addition to megaloblastosis the marrow in three of the patients had prominent ringed sideroblasts.

The usual tests for thiamine status are entirely normal. There was a slightly reduced α-ketoglutarate activity in fibroblast culture (174 pm/mg/min as compared to a mean of 240 in control cells). Treatment with 20 mg thiamine or more daily produces a reticulocyte response and a restoration of normal haemoglobin values (Fig. 14.6). Megaloblasts and ringed sideroblasts persist in the marrow after treatment. Relapse

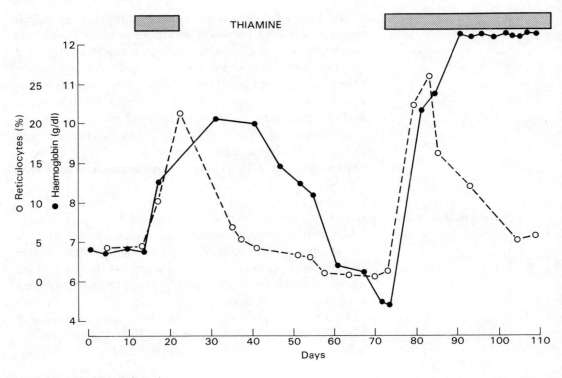

Fig. 14.6 The haematological response in thiamine-responsive megaloblastic anaemia to thiamine.

follows cessation of treatment and a further response ensues on re-treatment. There is no response to Cbl, folate and other haematinics. The severity of the diabetes is also ameliorated after thiamine treatment with a fall in fasting blood sugar and a flatter glucose tolerance curve [244].

The nature of the underlying lesion is not known.

Cellular uptake of 5-methyltetrahydrofolate

Impaired uptake (or retention) of labelled 5-methylfolate by phytohaemagglutinin-stimulated lymphocytes or red blood cells has been reported in two patients [246, 247].

The first [247] was a 36-year-old man with severe aplastic anaemia. He had a very strong family history of leukaemia, neutropenia and abnormal susceptibility to infection. Several family members had abnormal chromosomes. His aplastic anaemia remitted slowly on folic acid, first 5 mg daily and then 20 mg daily. His red cell folate level was 54 ng/ml after several months of folic acid (5 mg daily). The uptake of labelled methylfolate in stimulated lymphocytes (patient and family members) was less than in controls. Although this was attributed to impaired uptake, it could equally well have been due to impaired retention.

The second patient [248] has congenital dyserythropoietic anaemia and his red cells failed to take up labelled methylfolate as well as did control cells.

Folate deficiency in premature infants

Transfer of folate across the placenta is most active in the last weeks of pregnancy and the build-up of fetal stores is most evident after the 37th week. The mean red cell folate concentration in premature infants of 25–37 weeks gestation was 270 ng/ml red cells but in 135 full-term infants red cell folate averaged 340 ng/ml [248]. After birth the fall in red cell folate is greater in premature infants (Fig. 14.7) than in full-term ones [249]. The lowest red cell folates are reached at 7–10 weeks in smaller premature infants and at 11–12 weeks in larger infants. Serum folates reach their zenith at 4–8 weeks and it has been suggested that fetal folate stores are exhausted by 12 weeks [250] after which the newborn is dependent on dietary sources alone.

Human breast milk stored in the cold or frozen state shows a slow fall in folate content from 45 µg/l in the first week to 30 µg/l at 1 month, 25 µg/l at 2 months and 19 µg/l at 3 months. There is no change in folate content over 24 hours in the cold [251].

Heating of milk can have a deleterious effect on folate content if ascorbate levels are low. Thus pasteurization will reduce the ascorbate content. Reheating such milk can reduce the folate content from 54 to 10 µg/l. The supplementation of

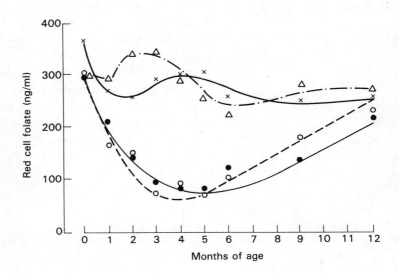

Fig. 14.7 Red cell folate levels in premature and full-term infants. •, 12 infants 28–30 weeks weighing 1030–1720 g; ○, 9 infants 32–35 weeks weighing 1820–2245 g; X, 35 full-term breast-fed infants; △, 10 infants 29–34 weeks weighing 1200–1750 g and receiving a folate supplement after day 14 to supply a folate intake of 50 µg daily.

powdered milk preparations with folate has redressed the problem of low folate content of such preparations.

Folate intake recommended by WHO for the first 3 months of life is 16 μg daily, between 3 and 6 months 24 μg daily and between 6 and 12 months 32 μg/day.

Megaloblastic haemopoiesis and anaemia in premature infants weighing 850–1150 g at birth and others weighing up to 1500 g and responding to folate, have been described [252, 253]. The cause was a combination of low folate stores and low folate content of re-heated milk feeds. The problem has disappeared with the general practice of giving a regular folate supplement to all premature infants for the first 12 weeks of life. Such folate-deficient infants failed to gain weight and their falling haemoglobin levels was not corrected by an iron supplement. A reticulocytosis and rising haemoglobin level followed folate therapy. It should be added that in malnourished populations a maternal folate supplement produced a significant increase in birth weight and produced a significant prolongation of pregnancy highlighting the importance too of folate deficiency as one of the causes of prematurity.

Disorders of folate metabolism without anaemia
Methylenetetrahydrofolate reductase deficiency

Methylenetetrahydrofolate reductase converts 5,10-CH_2H_4 — folate to 5-CH_3H_4folate. The CH_3-group that is formed is then passed on to homocysteine to form methionine, a pathway requiring both folate and Cbl coenzymes.

Deficiency of the enzyme results in a failure to make methylH$_4$folate and hence methionine in sufficient amount. There is homocystinuria. The clinical manifestations depend on the severity of the enzyme defect. The amount of methionine made by cells in fibroblast or lymphoid culture correlate well with the clinical state [254]:

	Methionine synthesized
Mildly affected	33–43% of normal
Moderately affected	10–11% of normal
Severely affected	4– 7% of normal

Mildly affected patients had severe CNS impairment with abnormal gait, spasticity, cerebellar ataxia and focal epilepsy. They tend to reach adult life. The moderatey affected patients in addition were mentally retarded; one patient exhibited schizophrenia-like behaviour [255]. Symptoms appear in early childhood and many die in the first or second decade. The severely affected present in early infancy with marked psychomotor retardation and developmental delay. They often die in infancy. Post-mortem may show thrombosis of vessels particularly in brain.

Methylene reductase activity in cell cultures is always low and very low in the severely affected infants (approximately 2% of the activity of control cultures). These patients all have homocystinuria. They are haematologically unaffected. Their serum folate level (normally $5\text{-}CH_3H_4PteGlu$) is very low. Their CSF folate is undetectable. Their red cell folate may be normal in amount but different in so far as it will support the growth of both *L.casei* and *S.faecalis* indicating that, unlike that in normal red cells, it is not methylH_4folate [256]. Their serum Cbl levels are normal. Methionine and S-adenosylmethionine levels were undetectable in some [257] but normal in others [256]. It is inherited as an autosomal recessive trait. Antenatal diagnosis can be made from amniocyte culture or chorionic villus sampling measuring methylene reductase activity [258, 259].

Some responses have been obtained with folic acid [255], methionine, folinic acid, pyridoxine, carnitine and Cbl [260] but the most promising substance is betaine which increases methionine synthesis from homocysteine by donating a CH_3-group [257, 261]. MethylH_4folate deserves a full clinical trial in this condition. Treatment with betaine results in a marked fall in homocystinuria and improvement in the mental state [261].

Formiminoglutamic aciduria   These patients excrete large amounts of formiminoglutamic acid in the urine. The first description was among Japanese patients in a psychiatric institution and all were severely retarded with cortical atrophy. They had normal serum folate levels. Subsequent cases were in children generally mildly retarded, some with hypotonia and delayed speech development but several had siblings excreting equally large amounts of formiminoglutamic acid who were clinically unaffected [262]. The enzyme activity of formiminotransferase in the liver and red blood cells was low in several patients. Marrows were normoblastic. Both folate and methionine were reported to reduce formiminoglutamic acid excretion [263, 436].

Hypersarcosinaemia   Increased levels of sarcosine in blood and urine results from a rare inborn error of metabolism. Although some individuals with this metabolic error are mildly retarded, in others it is an incidental finding.

Sarcosine is formed by the transfer of methyl groups from choline to yield betaine, dimethylglycine and sarcosine (methylglycine). It is also formed by methylation of glycine from S-adenosylmethionine [264]. Sarcosine is converted to glycine by oxidation of the methyl group to formaldehyde by sarcosine dehydrogenase. Similarly dimethylglycine is converted to sarcosine by methyl group oxidation by dimethyl glycine dehydrogenase. They are both mitochondrial enzymes. Folate coenzyme is involved as acceptor of the 1-carbon unit to yield 5,10-methyleneH$_4$PteGlu [50]. In hypersarcosinaemia there is impairment of sarcosine dehydrogenase. The folate coenzyme has been best characterized in relation to dimethylglycine dehydrogenase which contains tightly-bound tetrahydropteroylpentaglutamate [264]. Indeed this dimethylglycine dehydrogenase is one of the main folate-binding proteins in liver.

Chapter 15   Raised serum cobalamin levels

Raised serum Cbl levels are of themselves of limited diagnostic value and they occur in a variety of disease states. Other than when the raised Cbl level is due to acute hepatic damage as in acute hepatitis or the consequences of a large parenteral dose of Cbl, it is associated with an increase in Cbl-binding proteins in plasma usually R-binder but sometimes TCII.

Subjects of African negro stock have significantly higher serum Cbl levels than white subjects. This has been demonstrated in South Africa, Nigeria as well as in the UK and USA. A recent comparison among 49 subjects in each group was 546 ± 197 pg/ml (SD) for blacks in the USA and 382 ± 131 pg/ml for whites. The range for blacks was 195–943 and for whites 127–632 [265].

Liver damage releases Cbl into plasma and not surprisingly the highest serum Cbl levels are seen in patients with acute hepatic necrosis and in hepatic coma. In the early phase of acute hepatitis the serum Cbl level may be as high as 5000 pg/ml and levels are generally between three to eight times greater than normal. In patients with hepatic coma Cbl levels are 30–40 times greater than normal [7]. The levels return to normal over 3–4 weeks with recovery. It is assumed that the high levels are the result of the release of Cbl from necrosed hepatocytes.

In hepatic cirrhosis the serum Cbl level ranged from 317 to 1306 pg/ml (mean 759) and was somewhat lower in biliary cirrhosis, 203–928 pg/ml with a mean of 468. In all these patients there was increased urinary excretion of Cbl indicating increased unbound Cbl in plasma [266].

An interesting situation occurs in patients with primary carcinoma of the liver where the tumour may produce an R-type Cbl binder in large amounts which is excreted into plasma and leads to very high plasma Cbl levels. Thus among 37 patients seen in Thailand 34 had raised serum Cbl levels ranging from 440 to 4570 pg/ml with a mean of 1730 [267]. The

133

serum unsaturated Cbl-binding capacity was greatly increased and in ten out of 107 patients who had high Cbl levels ranged from 39 to 379 ng/ml (normal 0.7–1.6) [268]. In one patient the tumour contained ten times more Cbl binder than did normal liver in the same patient [269]. In some the R-binder was considered to have an increased sialic acid content and this resulted in slow plasma clearance so that the R-binder accumulated in plasma [270]. The abnormal protein (and Cbl level) rises with progression of the hepatoma and falls with response to chemotherapy.

Occasionally high serum Cbl levels are present in patients with disseminated neoplasia from the stomach, colon or bronchus. The R-binder may be complexed into a larger macromolecule in some patients [271].

The other major group of patients with raised serum Cbl levels are those with myeloproliferative disorders most notably chronic myelocytic leukaemia. Over 90% of patients with chronic myelocytic leukaemia in relapse have serum Cbl levels above 2000 pg/ml and may exceed 14 000 pg/ml. It is generally considered that the leukocytes are the source of the increased Cbl binder and generally the level fluctuates with the state of the disease falling with remission and rising in relapse. Increased serum Cbl levels also occur in juvenile chronic myelocytic leukaemia and in the hypereosinophil syndrome. The Cbl level may fall in the blast cell crisis [272].

The serum Cbl level in 22 patients with untreated polycythaemia rubra vera was 984 ± 1072 pg/ml (s.d.). The serum Cbl level was equally high in chronic myelofibrosis (mean 1082 ± 623 pg/ml) but was normal in spurious or stress polycythaemia. Twenty-two out of 49 patients with myelofibrosis had serum Cbl levels above the normal range [273].

Increased levels of TCII have been reported in disseminated lupus, dermatomyositis, autoimmune haemolytic anaemia and renal transplant patients [437] as well as in Gaucher's disease [274] although the serum Cbl level is generally normal.

Increased serum Cbl levels occur in cystic fibrosis [275] and in renal failure [276].

Chapter 16   Nutritional folate deficiency

Nutritional folate deficiency may be the sole cause of megaloblastic anaemia but more commonly is one of several factors that lead to a negative folate balance. Thus an inadequate dietary intake may accompany alcoholism, pregnancy, a chronic haemolytic state, chronic myelofibrosis or medication with anticonvulsant drugs and together be responsible for a megaloblastic anaemia.

In the absence of these additional factors nutritional megaloblastic anaemia can be diagnosed only when other causes of megaloblastic anaemia have been excluded and when careful dietary assessment confirms a very low dietary folate content.

The second National Health and Nutrition Examination survey (NHANES II) in the USA carried out between 1976 and 1980 noted that folate nutrition may be sub-optimal in pregnant women, elderly persons and adolescents of low socio-economic status. The frequency of folate deficiency as assessed by low red cell folates (Table 16.1) reached 8% in adult males and 13% in premenopausal women. Dietary folate has been shown to correlate well with red cell folate but not with serum folate [277]. A similar frequency of low red cell folates to that noted in the NHANES study has been reported by others — 12% among elderly patients admitted to hospital in England [278]; 10% among elderly people in residential homes in Norway [279]; and 8% among elderly people living in the com-

Table 16.1 Percentage of subjects with RBC folate levels below 140 ng/ml in the US population (NHANES II)

Age (years)	Males		Females	
	No. examined	% low	No. examined	% low
0.5– 9	243	2	201	2
10–19	178	5	173	8
20–44	299	8	389	13
45–74	503	8	439	4

135

munity in Wales [280]. Much higher frequencies of reduced red cell folate levels have been reported — 22% among elderly hospital patients in Montreal [281] and even 60% in Florida. Some of these very high frequencies must raise questions about the technical adequacy of the studies. A value based on 14 reports suggested a frequency of low red cell folate of 8.7% for elderly subjects at home and 18% for institutionalized patients [282].

Measurement of dietary folate in Sweden indicated a daily intake of 366 µg (range 295–531) in men aged 25–60 years and an intake of 153 µg per day (range 103–239) in men aged 68–70 years. The corresponding figures for women were 129 µg folate per day (range 84–239) in the 25–60-year age group and 125 µg folate per day (range 49–120) in the 68–70-year age group [283]. The great majority of subjects with low red cell folates are not anaemic but must be at greater risk of developing megaloblastosis than those with normal red cell folate levels.

However, liver folate concentrations measured in samples collected at autopsy in Canada did not substantiate a significant incidence of folate deficiency. Indeed only two out of 560 samples gave low values and there was no trend to lower values among the elderly [282]. This correlates with the relative rarity of megaloblastic anaemia due to simple nutritional folate deficiency in developed countries.

The sequence of events in experimental nutritional folate deficiency is an early fall in serum folate evident in the second week but the fall in red cell folate only appears after 5 weeks [67, 284]. Liver folate concentration falls steadily but macrocytosis and megaloblastosis do not develop for at least 18 weeks [67] (Fig. 16.1).

The recognition of megaloblastic haemopoiesis has been discussed elsewhere. Since pernicious anaemia is the likeliest diagnosis in the older patient, adequate investigation to exclude this and other disorders is required before embarking on folate therapy. However, even in the absence of an overt megaloblastic process, treatment in those who have laboratory evidence of folate deficiency can be beneficial. Responses to folate in ten elderly patients who had a variety of neurological disorders were reported. These include a psychotic patient with spastic paraplegia who returned home ambulent and well after folate [285]. A French group treated 50 unselected, elderly folate-deficient patients with folate and reported a significant improvement in 30–40% using a self-

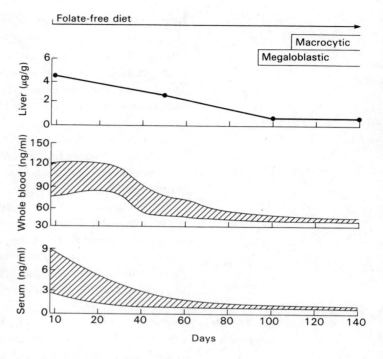

Fig. 16.1 Studies on seven patients with neoplasia on a folate 'free' diet. Serum and liver folate levels fall at a steady rate but there is a lag of about 30 days before the red cell folate falls. The mean MCV rose from 88 to 102 fl after 110 days. Megaloblastic marrows were noted after day 90. Liver biopsy data on one patient is shown [284].

rating scale and neuropsychiatric assessment [286]. It is clearly important to ensure an adequate dietary folate intake in elderly subjects.

Nutritional folate deficiency may also occur in the very young — premature infants (Chapter 14) and in those on artificial diets that do not contain adequate folate such as those used in treatment of phenylketonuria and maple-syrup disease [7]. The clinical experience is that megaloblastic anaemia due to uncomplicated nutritional folate deficiency does not occur in teenage subjects in developed countries.

Developing countries

Nutritional folate deficiency is far more prevalent in Africa, Asia and South America than in developed countries. Not surprisingly hard data are not readily available.

Red cell folates, among subjects in Benin (Central Africa), were below 160 ng/ml in 26% of adult males, in 30% of women of childbearing age and in 34% of post-menopausal women. Only 6% of children aged 6–14 years had low red cell folates but below 6 years the frequency was 25–31% [287]. Among 254 Algerian women of childbearing age 37% had red cell folate values below 100 ng/ml [288].

In Thailand it has been reported that the diet is normally

rich in folates and red cell folate values were mostly normal
[289]. In the Dominican Republic (West Indies) red cell folates
among 42 villagers were all normal [290]. Studies among
immigrants in the USA showed that less than 1% of 300
Mexican children had a low red cell folate [291]. Among Asian
Indian immigrants to Canada 12.1% of the males had a red
cell folate below 140 ng/ml as did 33.3% of the females [292].
In Scotland red cell folate levels below 100 ng/ml were found
in 2.8% of 177 Asian Indian and Pakistani children, in 7% of
African children, 2.5% of Chinese children and in 5.2% of
Scottish children [293].

Reports of megaloblastic anaemia due to presumed nutritional megaloblastic anaemia [7] and a relatively high incidence of megaloblastic anaemia in pregnancy in developing
countries indicate a relatively high prevalence of nutritional
folate deficiency even if this is not always substantiated by
population studies on folate status.

Scurvy and folate
deficiency

Ascorbate and folate are both heat labile and destroyed by
oxidation. They occur in the same types of food and are both
water soluble. A diet deficient in one is likely to be deficient
in the other. Furthermore, ascorbate in food protects folate
from oxidation and loss of ascorbate makes the folate vulner-
able. This occurs in preparing a milk formula for infant feeding when ascorbate is lost in the initial warming and the folate
lost in the second heating before giving the milk. A large
minority of patients with clinical scurvy have either a megaloblastic marrow or an overt megaloblastic anaemia.

Scorbutic patients who are normoblastic respond only to
ascorbate. Mildly megaloblastic patients may show a small
response to folate but a larger response when ascorbate is
added. When megaloblastic anaemia is more pronounced an
initial response to folate is followed by a second reticulocytosis with ascorbate. If ascorbate is given as the first line of
treatment a complete response may occur [294–296]. Unfor-
tunately, data on red cell folate levels are not available.

Production of scurvy in monkeys by feeding cows' milk
resulted in combined ascorbate and folate deficiency. Livers
had very low levels of both vitamins. Adding only folate to
the diet precipitated clinical scurvy. When scurvy was severe,
the marrow became megaloblastic and then responded to
either folate or ascorbate. It was concluded that ascorbate
deficiency increased folate requirements but there was no
special relationship between the two [297]. Similarly in man it

was suggested that when megaloblastic anaemia and scurvy coincided there was simultaneous deficiency of folate and ascorbate [296]. In the guinea-pig ascorbate deficiency did not affect tissue folate levels [298].

Under some circumstances ascorbate added to Cbl can destroy the Cbl [299]. This is unlikely to occur in a clinical context. *In vitro* conversion of Cbl to CNCbl protects against reduction by ascorbate [300].

Chapter 17 Folate deficiency in pregnancy

There is an increased requirement for both iron and folate in pregnancy. If this increased requirement cannot be met from body stores and the diet, deficiency ensues.

Physiological changes in pregnancy

Normal pregnancy is accompanied by an expansion of the plasma volume by about 1000 ml and by an expansion of the red cell volume by about 300 ml. The greater expansion of plasma volume results in dilution of red cells so that their concentration per unit of blood falls. Thus the mean haemoglobin falls from 13.5 g/dl in the non-pregnant state to 12.5 g/dl at 15 weeks of pregnancy and 12.0 g/dl at 30 weeks of pregnancy. Thereafter there is some haemoconcentration so that the mean haemoglobin at 38 weeks in 12.8 g/dl. At 30 weeks the range for haemoglobin is 10.0–14.5 g/dl.

At the same time there is an increase in the MCV which at term on average is 4 fl greater than in early pregnancy. In some women the increase in the MCV is much greater being as much as 20 fl, so that the MCV at term is about 105 fl. This is not influenced by folate supplements and the marrow remains normoblastic. Iron deficiency as well as β-thalassaemia trait prevents a full increase in the MCV [301, 302]. These values return to pre-pregnancy levels 6 weeks postnatally.

Iron

In pregnancy iron is required for the fetus (300 mg), the placenta (50 mg), the increase of maternal red cell mass (450 mg) and for meeting normal basal iron losses by the mother (240 mg). At delivery maternal blood loss equates to a loss of 250 mg of iron. After delivery the return to a reduced pre-pregnancy red cell mass makes available some 450 mg of iron. Thus the total additional amount of iron that has to be found during pregnancy is about 1000 mg. This should be set against the background of a total iron content of about 2500–3000 mg for an adult woman and a normal iron absorption of 1–2 mg daily. Iron absorption increases in pregnancy to about

140

4 mg day. However, at about the 22nd week of pregnancy, daily iron requirement is 5 mg increasing steadily to 10 mg per day after the 36th week. Thus iron requirements are too high to be covered by physiological absorption from a western-type diet and even less so from a vegetarian diet where iron availability is low. Iron requirements have to be met from iron stores which are often low or even absent and when stores are exhausted maternal iron deficiency ensues as the fetus continues to take priority in iron supply. Only an iron supplement can ensure that the pregnant woman remains iron sufficient.

Folate   It is not possible to do similar calculations in relation to folate status. An increased folate requirement in pregnancy arises from the role of folate in synthesis of nucleosides for DNA replication. The increased cell division accompanying expansion of the mother's red cell mass, development of the placenta, growth of the uterus and of the fetus require increased amounts of folate, as does the active transfer of folate to the fetus, particularly in late pregnancy [303]. This increased requirement is evident by the 20th week of pregnancy when there is more rapid clearance of small injected doses of folate from plasma to tissues. Thereafter requirement continues to increase being maximal in the last trimester. At the same time there is increased loss of folate into the urine, possibly due to a lowered renal threshold. The renal loss averages 14 µg per day as compared to 4.2 µg daily in non-pregnant women and 3.5 µg daily in the puerperium. In some women urinary loss exceeded 50 µg daily [304] in pregnancy and this too is a significant factor in producing a negative folate balance.

The increased folate requirement has to be met from the diet and where the diet supplies an above average amount of folate, indeed, folate status is maintained. This, however, is not the usual state of affairs and most women are in negative folate balance.

Cobalamin   Serum cobalamin levels fall in pregnancy and at term the levels are below 170 pg/ml in about 5% of healthy women. Low levels are more frequent in those who are megaloblastic. The explanation for the low Cbl level is that dietary cobalamin is shunted to the placenta and fetus particularly in the latter weeks of pregnancy. Maternal stores of Cbl are about 3000 µg; that of the fetus is about 50 µg. The events of pregnancy therefore have no significant impact on maternal Cbl status

Table 17.1 Mean cobalamin and folate levels in paired maternal and newborn bloods [303]

	Mother	Cord blood
Serum Cbl (pg/ml)	296	572
Serum folate (ng/ml)	3.2	17.1
Red cell folate (ng/ml)	149	325

and the serum Cbl level in pregnancy should be ignored. It is even possible for a woman with early pernicious anaemia to have a normal pregnancy with a normal outcome and the pointer to any problem is megaloblastic anaemia due to Cbl deficiency in the child presenting several months after birth (Chapter 12). Serum Cbl levels return to their pre-pregnancy levels in the puerperium.

Serum Cbl and folate levels as well as red cell folate levels are much higher in cord blood than in maternal blood (Table 17.1) indicating active transfer of these nutrients across the placenta.

Folate status in pregnancy

In the USA 13% of randomly-selected women of childbearing age have evidence of sub-clinical folate deficiency in so far as they have low red cell folate levels (NHANES II study). It is thus not surprising that 16% of women at their first visit to an antenatal clinic in New York had low red cell folate levels [305]. In London 10% of women had reduced red cell folates at first clinic attendance [306] as did 16% in Brazil [307]. In Nigeria the corresponding figure was 31% [308] in women seen before the 26th week.

The red cell folate falls throughout pregnancy indicating a negative maternal folate balance. Thus in London red cell folate levels at 12, 24, 36 weeks and the puerperium were 317, 302, 288 and 252 ng/ml, respectively [306]. In Paris red cell folate at 3, 6 and 9 months of pregnancy were 314, 266 and 213 ng/ml, respectively [309]. Between 24 and 32% of women have reduced red cell folate levels at term. In a French study 50% of women had red cell folate levels below 150 ng/ml at 6 months [310]. On the other hand in Denmark and Australia red cell folate levels were maintained during pregnancy. This might indicate an adequate dietary folate intake during pregnancy but may on the other hand be due to drifts in folate assay procedures. Small changes in folate levels are best assessed if all samples are stored and assayed together in a single batch. A correlation between dietary folate intake in pregnancy and red cell folate has been noted; the red cell folate averaged 202 ng/ml in those taking less than 113 µg folate daily and 254 ng/ml in those taking more than 176 µg folate daily [311]. In Nigeria 85% of primigravidae had low red cell folate levels at term [308] as did 45% in Benin [312].

Serum folate too falls in pregnancy. In a large study in Aberdeen values at presentation, 30 weeks, 36 weeks and the puerperium were 6.6, 5.2, 4.5 and 3.7 ng/ml, respectively [313]. Expansion of plasma volume was considered a factor in the fall in serum folate. Low levels occur in between 15 and 54% of women in different series [7].

Urinary formiminoglutamic acid excretion is a particularly poor test of folate status in pregnancy as histidine, the precursor of formiminoglutamic acid, is handled differently at different stages of pregnancy. A significant amount of histidine is lost in the urine due to a lowered renal threshold in pregnancy and megaloblastic anaemia in pregnancy can occur with normal formiminoglutamic acid excretion [7].

Anaemia in pregnancy

The major cause of anaema in pregnancy is iron deficiency. Even in developed countries this will develop in about one-third of pregnancies if iron supplements are not given.

The frequency of anaemia due to folate deficiency, in the absence of a folate supplement, relates to the effort made in its detection. There is no difficulty in recognition of overt megaloblastic anaemia but this is uncommon in developed countries, although relatively common under poor nutritional circumstances. The difficulty in recognition of milder examples stems from the presence of underlying iron deficiency so that microcytosis rather than macrocytosis is present, the megaloblastic process appears late in pregnancy, and hypersegmented neutrophils can be due to iron deficiency as well as to folate deficiency.

The presence of small numbers of macrocytes in a microcyte red cell population in the blood film is suggestive but final diagnosis requires marrow aspiration. Red cell folates are still within the normal range in one-third of women who have megaloblastic marrows in pregnancy [7]. These red cell folate levels are falling as new red cells (macrocytes) will have a very low folate content. But the dilution of red cells of higher folate content by red cells with low folate content has not yet reached a point in a third of patients where the total red cell folate is low.

In the absence of folate supplementation evidence of megaloblastic anaemia was noted in 2.8% of 3199 pregnant women in England by examination of the peripheral blood [314]. More assiduous scrutiny of peripheral blood suggested a diagnosis of megaloblastic anaemia in 6–12% of pregnant women in Glasgow and Liverpool and in 24% of women in Malaysia [315].

There is however a remarkably high frequency of megaloblastic haemopoiesis based on 'routine' marrow examination. No less than 25% of all pregnant women near term have megaloblastic marrows as reported in London, Montreal, Johannesburg and Texas [315]. In Ireland and Nigeria the frequency of megaloblastic marrows was 30% and in South India 54–60% [315].

There is often a seasonal incidence to megaloblastic anaemia in pregnancy, being highest at the end of the season of the year when fresh vegetables are least available. Megaloblastic anaemia is some eight times more frequent among twin than among singleton pregnancies and is more common in multigravidae than in primigravidae. There is a tendency for megaloblastic anaemia to recur in a second pregnancy. These data imply a greater requirement for folate in twin pregnancies and a continuation of an inadequate diet from one pregnancy to the next. Iron deficiency occurs in the same women who are megaloblastic and reflects dietary deficiency of both iron and folate.

Diagnosis is usually made in the last few weeks of pregnancy in half the patients and in the puerperium in the other half. Where there is an additional factor increasing folate requirement such as a haemolytic anaemia, megaloblastic anaemia may present as early as the second trimester.

Occasional patients present with purpura, a low platelet count, often urinary tract infection, hypersegmented neutrophils but few other changes in the peripheral blood which shows features of iron deficiency. Their marrows, however, show very severe megaloblastic changes [316, 317].

In all cases megaloblastic anaemia in pregnancy is due to folic acid deficiency.

Effects of folate deficiency

A variety of consequences have been attributed to folate deficiency in pregnancy in addition to megaloblastic anaemia but most have not been supported by better planned studies. Only two merit more serious consideration, the development of neural tube defects and prematurity.

The case for folate deficiency in very early pregnancy as a factor in causing neural tube defects rests on data from trials in which folate supplements given before conception to women who had already had an affected infant, reduced the incidence of neural tube defect. In one study 1% of mothers in the vitamin-supplemented group had a child with a neural tube defect as compared to 4% in mothers not receiving a supplement [318]. In a second report there were no examples of neural tube defect in a group given 4 mg folic acid a day before and during early pregnancy but six examples among those not taking the supplement or taking a placebo [319].

The importance of folic acid deficiency as one of the factors responsible for low birth weight infants and prematurity was demonstrated in a well-controlled trial [320]. The study involved a well-nourished Caucasian group and an African group whose staple diet was boiled maize. Each supplemented group of 50–60 pregnant women received either iron (200 mg), or iron and folate (5 mg) or iron and folate + cobalamin (50 µg). The birth weights were recorded (Table 17.2). The supplements made no difference to birth weights in the better nourished white subjects. Africans given only iron gave birth to 19 infants weighing less than 2270 g (5 lbs). When a folate supplement was given the number of low birth weight infants fell to four and the mean birth weight for the group rose from 2466 to 2798 g. The addition of cobalamin did not have a significant effect. These data have been confirmed [315]. Folate supplementation prolonged the period of gestation by 1 week [321] and increased placental size from 456 g in iron-supplemented women to 517 g in iron and folate-supplemented women [322] suggesting that the increased birth weight is due to better fetal nutrition. In Gambia the beneficial effects of a dietary supplement was only seen in the wet season when there was a shortage of food and not in the dry season when women were adequately nourished [323]. In Denmark, however, a 5 mg daily folate supplement led to an increase in both birth weight and placental size [324]

Table 17.2 Effect of iron, folate and cobalamin supplements in pregnancy on birth weight and prematurity [320]

Newborn weight (g)	Caucasian			African		
	Iron	Iron + Folate	Iron + Folate + Cbl	Iron	Iron + Folate	Iron + Folate + Cbl
<2270	2	2	2	19	4	1
>2270	50	60	56	44	61	54
Mean	3114	3164	3110	2466	2798	2871

despite the claim that maternal red cell folates did not fall during pregnancy [315].

Attempts have been made to correlate folate deficiency with increased incidence of abruptio placentae, toxaemia, abortion, stillbirth and congenital malformations. Other than possibly neural tube defects a relation has not been established.

Prophylaxis with iron and folate in pregnancy

The high frequency of these deficiencies and the consequences on mother and child, has led to the wide acceptance that routine provision of iron/folate supplements in pregnancy should be the norm. This view was endorsed by an international specialist forum hosted by WHO in Geneva in 1988. Thirty mg iron daily will prevent the development of anaemia in pregnancy [315]. Folate requirement has been determined by the amount needed to prevent a fall in red cell folate throughout pregnancy. Total daily folate intake to achieve this is of the order of 260 µg daily. As the dietary folate varies from 60 µg daily to more than 200 µg, the supplement should contain at least 200 µg folate. Thus the desirable supplement in pregnancy should supply between 30 and 100 mg iron and 200 µg pteroyglutamic acid taken once daily throughout pregnancy [315]. This will meet the requirements of those taking the poorest diet although supplying rather more than is required for those taking a reasonably good diet. In Sweden it was found that whole blood folate continued to fall with a 50 µg folate supplement daily during pregnancy but rose by about 20% with 100 µg folate daily, by 60% with 200 µg daily and by 100% with 500 µg folate daily [325]. In London a daily folate supplement of 100 µg folate produced a rise in red cell folate during the second trimester which stabilized in the third trimester whereas red cell folate continued to fall in those receiving only iron [306] (Fig. 17.1). The wide use of iron/folate prophylaxis has made anaemia in pregnancy a rarity other than in those not receiving antenatal care. Recent suggestions to limit prophylaxis to those women with serum ferritin levels, say below 50 µg/l [326], are likely to exclude only a minority of pregnant women and these will require careful surveillance to ensure that they do not develop anaemia.

Lactation

The frequency of megaloblastosis in pregnancy ranges between 25 and 60%. In the puerperium, with declining demands for folate, normoblastic haemopoiesis is restored as more folate is available to the mother. In a few however the demands of

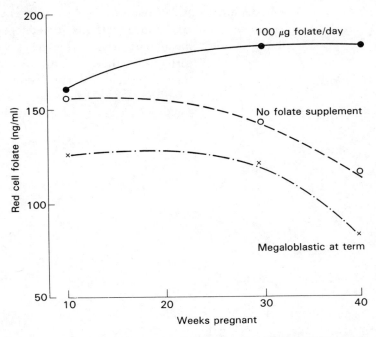

Fig. 17.1 One group of 105 women received iron and 100 µg folate daily and a second group of 101 women received iron only. The red cell folate fell in the group receiving only iron but rose in the first trimester in the folate supplemented group and stabilized after the 30th week of pregnancy. Eighteen out of the 206 women were found to have megaloblastic marrows at term. These not only had the lowest red cell folates at term but also had lower red cell folates in early pregnancy indicating underlying nutritional folate deficiency antedating their pregnancy.

lactation combined with a poor diet allows a folate-deficient state to persist. Human milk after the second month of lactation contains 25 µg folate/l and with a secretion of 700 ml involves a loss of about 20 µg folate daily to the mother. In lactation a small supplemental dose of folate (100 µg daily) leads to an increase in breast milk folate without any increase in maternal serum folate and this remains true in those women whose folate deficiency was accompanied by an overt megaloblastic anaemia [327]. Thus folate is preferentialy shunted to secretion into milk. Milk contains an avid folate binder that potentiates transfer of serum folate into milk. In Burma only five of 56 women were diagnosed as having megaloblastic anaemia in pregnancy and the remainder presented with megaloblastic anaemia 2–18 months after delivery [328]. As in pregnancy it has been estimated that 200–300 µg folate daily is required during lactation [328].

Increased folate requirement   An increased folate requirement is present in women who take anticonvulsants for epilepsy, in those with a chronic haemolytic state (sickle cell anaemia, hereditary spherocytosis) and in those with malaria. In these, pregnancy results in folate deficiency and megaloblastic anaemia in the second trimester of pregnancy rather than the third trimester and folate prophylaxis should supply 500 µg folate daily rather than 260 µg.

Chapter 18   Folate and alcohol

Not only is there a strong association between megaloblastic anaemia and excessive alcohol consumption but undisclosed alcohol abuse is not infrequently the explanation of an otherwise puzzling megaloblastic anaemia.

Metabolism of alcohol

About 80% of ingested ethanol is metabolized by the liver, about 10% is metabolized in extrahepatic sites including bone marrow and the rest is excreted. Ethanol is oxidized to acetaldehyde mainly by cytosolic enzymes termed alcohol dehydrogenases but some by a microsomal ethanol-oxidizing system (MEOS). This latter system involves oxidases located in the smooth endoplasmic reticulum which proliferates in response to alcohol exposure and this is responsible for enzyme induction by alcohol.

Acetaldehyde, the product of ethanol metabolism, is more reactive chemically than ethanol and may be responsible for many effects associated with alcohol. It is oxidized by acetaldehyde dehydrogenases to acetate.

Amount of ethanol

It is difficult to set down minimal acceptable levels of alcohol consumption. The relative risk of harmful effects from alcohol was six times greater in those taking 40–60 g ethanol daily as compared to those taking 0–20 g daily. At 60–80 g daily the risk was 14 times greater [401]. Generally, 60 g ethanol daily is excessive; 7–9 g ethanol is contained in 280 ml beer, 120 ml wine, 60 ml sherry or 24 ml spirits.

The patients

Studies have been made in two groups of patients. One group consumes alcohol at the expense of other food. In the US these so-called 'skid-row' alcoholics have formed the basis of studies on the effects of severe alcoholism, patients often having been admitted to hospital in alcoholic coma. By contrast other studies have involved subjects taking excessive alcohol while generally taking adequate nutrition and remain-

149

ing integrated into their families and communities. The findings in these two groups are very different.

Effect of alcohol on haemopoiesis

In general there are two kinds, the direct toxic effect of ethanol (or its metabolic products) on developing haemopoietic cells and perhaps their progenity in the peripheral blood and, secondly, effects that are added to this due to folate deficiency, which is largely nutritional in origin.

The direct toxic effects of alcohol

Growth of erythroid colonies from marrow progenitor cells is suppressed by concentrations of alcohol present *in vivo*. Acetaldehyde is a more potent suppressor than ethanol. Pluripotential stem cells are not affected and granulocyte progenitors are more resistant than erythroid progenitors [329]. Megakaryocyte precursors too are resistant to ethanol but the mature megakaryocyte is affected as demonstrated by impaired protein synthesis.

The effect of alcohol on marrow progenitor cells may be the explanation of the hypocellularity of marrow in chronic alcoholics and this is reversed on alcohol withdrawal. Often there are no recognizable abnormalities in marrow morphology. In those taking large quantities of alcohol, particularly 'skid-row' alcoholics, changes are present in more than half the patients. These changes consist of megaloblastic erythroblasts; vacuolation most notably in the cytoplasm of proerythroblasts but also occurring in immature granulocytes and sometimes present over the nucleus; and of impaired haemoglobin formation manifest as ringed sideroblasts. Thus in 26 US patients admitted to hospital because of alcoholism, 11 had delirium tremens, eight were megaloblastic and 14 had multiple vacuoles. In another study in the USA involving severe alcoholics with liver disease ringed sideroblasts were present in the marrow of 24 out of 33 patients. A Swiss study on 30 patients admitted for a detoxification course noted megaloblasts in 28, ringed sideroblasts in 28, and vacuolated proerythroblasts in all 30. Multinuclear erythroblasts were seen in 17 patients and iron granules in plasma cells in 29 [330].

In contrast marrows in 57 patients in London mostly taking an adequate diet and taking more than 80 g ethanol daily showed megaloblasts in 27 (47%), vacuolation in nine (16%) and scanty ringed sideroblasts in four (7%) [331].

The commonest change in the peripheral blood is macrocytosis. A raised MCV in a patient with a normal haemoglobin level suggests a diagnosis of alcoholism in the first instance. The frequency with which macrocytosis is recorded depends on the views held on the normal range for the MCV. When the upper limit was set at 100 fl only 42% of 118 US alcoholic patients were macrocytic [332]. The frequency for macrocytosis when the upper limit of the MCV was between 92 and 94 fl was 80% [331] (Fig. 18.1). Despite uncertainties about the level of the cut-off point for the MCV, it has proved to be a valuable screen for alcohol excess in clinical practice and comparable in sensitivity to serum gamma-glutamyl transpeptidase. With an MCV of 95 as the upper limit, macrocytosis was present in 70% of alcoholics with liver disease and in 23% of non-alcoholics with liver disease. Macrocytosis was present in 86% of the women and 63% of the men. An MCV above 100 fl was present in 50% of alcoholics but only 3% of non-alcoholics [333]. Macrocytosis was identified in 3% of 8000 employees of a US insurance company. Of 17 recalled

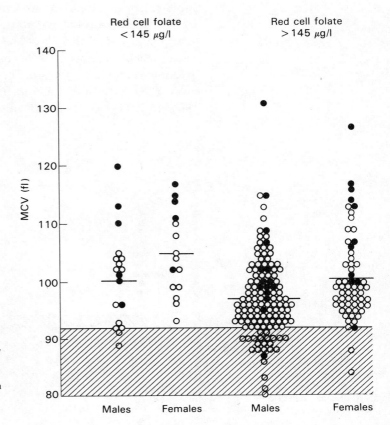

Fig. 18.1 The MCV in alcoholics taking more than 80 g ethanol daily grouped in relation to sex and their folate status. Macrocytosis is present in the majority of patients and is not related to a low red cell folate level. Megaloblastosis on marrow aspiration (●) is present in both those with low and with normal red cell folate levels. Those with a higher MCV are more likely to be megaloblastic.

for further examination, all but one consumed excess alcohol [334].

Scanning electron microscope examination of red cells from alcoholics may show two to three large indentations. Stomatocytes are not uncommon in blood films. Changes of a megaloblastic anaemia due to folate deficiency may occur. A dimorphic blood picture may be present in patients with megaloblastosis and in these there are large numbers of ringed sideroblasts in the marrow [335]. Rarely a spur cell anaemia may be present accompanied by transient hypobetalipoproteinaemia and due to accompanying liver disease [336].

Anaemia is variable and was present in only 11 of 84 patients in the UK [331] and in about 50% of malnourished alcoholics in the USA taking more than 100 g ethanol daily, 19% of whom died [332]. Leukopenia was present in only 6% of patients and thrombocytopenia in 55% [332].

The evidence that these changes are due to the direct toxic effect of alcohol or to its products rests with the relatively rapid disappearance of all these phenomena on alcohol withdrawal alone. Alcohol withdrawal causes a reticulocytosis reaching a peak after 7 days and, where there is uncomplicated anaemia, to a rise in haemoglobin. In the absence of splenomegaly the platelets increase and the white cell count rises. Megaloblasts and abnormal vacuoles are gone after 5 days and sideroblasts largely disappear within 7 days and

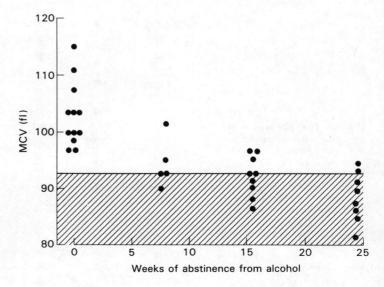

Fig. 18.2 Unlike other abnormalities in the blood and marrow which disappear within 1–2 weeks of alcohol withdrawal, the large red blood cells survive more than 100 days and hence a normal MCV after alcohol withdrawal is not restored until this time had elapsed.

disappear in all within 12 days. Macrocytes however disappear after 100 or more days (Fig. 18.2).

In addition to reversal on alcohol withdrawal the blood changes are present in those who have normal folate status as well as those who are folate deficient (Fig. 18.1). This includes megaloblastosis [331]. The addition of folate does not prevent alcohol producing megaloblastic changes within days of its administration [337]. Finally the deoxyuridine suppression test on marrows from alcoholic patients is normal despite megaloblastosis, an indication that the megaloblastosis does not arise through impairment of Cbl–folate pathways [338].

Cobalamin metabolism in alcoholics

There is a tendency for alcoholic patients to have somewhat raised serum Cbl levels. This is generally ascribed to the release of Cbl from damaged hepatocytes. Alcoholics without liver damage had a mean serum Cbl level of 317 pg/ml, with mild liver damage 417 pg/ml, moderate liver damage 1014 pg/ml and with severe liver damage 1507 pg/ml [339]. A low Cbl level in an alcoholic should be investigated in the same way as a low Cbl level in any other patient and may be due to accompanying pernicious anaemia or secondary to a folate-deficient megaloblastic anaemia.

Folate metabolism in alcoholics

In the UK, one-third of alcoholics seen in the medical department of a hospital had folate deficiency as defined by a low serum, red cell and liver folate concentration [331]. In common with other reports, the main causes were an inadequate diet and alcohol in the form of spirits. Beer drinkers have a lower incidence of folate deficiency due to the significant folate content of beer.

Other mechanisms for the development of folate deficiency have been postulated but either remain unproven or their significance is uncertain.

Impaired intestinal absorption is demonstrable in patients taking large amounts of alcohol particularly so-called binge drinkers. There is a smaller rise in blood folate levels after an oral dose of folate in alcoholics than in controls and there is reduced absorption of folate perfused through a gut segment *in vivo* [340]. Impaired absorption of cobalamin and other water-soluble vitamins have also been demonstrated. The importance of this in producing a negative folate balance is uncertain. The action appears to be an inhibition of carrier-mediated transport by an effect on the enterocyte membrane [341].

An interruption in the enterohepatic circulation of folate in alcohol-treated rats with failure of excretion into bile was suggested but not confirmed by others [342].

Alcohol causes an increased loss of folate into the urine in rats and monkeys; it is not known whether this occurs in man [343]. There is no evidence for increased folate catabolism [342]. There is no impairment in the hepatic uptake of folate and its conversion into polyglutamates [344].

Volunteers taking large amounts of alcohol show a fall in serum folate starting a few hours after the peak alcohol blood level in reached and the level is restored after alcohol withdrawal [342]. The mechanism has not been established although urinary loss, failure of tissue release or increased catabolism have all been explored with negative or contradictory results. A dose of diphenylhydantoin has a similar effect and has been ascribed to increased catabolism of folate following enzyme induction.

Methionine synthetase activity in the liver of rats fed alcohol declines by about one-third and there is an increase in betaine-homocysteine methyltransferase [345].

Experimental studies in monkeys

In folate replete monkeys receiving 50% of their energy requirements as alcohol for 2 years there was a fall in hepatic folate from 6.0 µg/g in controls to 4.2 µg/g. When [^{3}H]-labelled folate was given there was reduced incorporation into the liver of alcohol-fed monkeys and increased excretion of the label into the urine. The distribution of folate analogues in the liver was unaltered. In animals studied for 4 years increased faecal loss of folate was noted [346]. Thus increased loss of folate was found.

A second study involved monkeys fed a folate-free diet for 1 year. These animals had mild anaemia, macrocytosis and megaloblastic marrows. One group received alcohol supplying 30% of energy requirements. The effects of the alcohol were minor; the alcohol-fed monkeys had higher urinary formiminoglutamic acid excretion but absorbed folate normally. However, loss of folate was via faeces rather than urine in the alcohol group suggesting impaired reabsorption of biliary folate [347].

Experimental studies in man

Heroic studies have been set up in 'volunteers', usually alcoholic patients recovering from hospitalization and given further alcohol [337]. These have shown that alcohol depresses haemopoiesis with a fall in reticulocytes and haemoglobin levels and a rise in serum iron level. These are reversed on alcohol withdrawal. A fall in serum folate has been mentioned. Folate-deficient subjects became megaloblastic on alcohol exposure but this effect could not be obtained when they had received adequate amounts of folate.

Iron, alcohol and folate   Alcohol given with iron substantially increases the amount of iron absorbed [348]. Some alcoholics have substantially increased iron stores with considerable elevation of serum ferritin. However, using rabbits it was found that alcohol augmented iron absorption only when they were folate deficient [349]. It is not known if this also applies in man.

Alcohol and cell membranes   The multitude of defects associated with alcohol suggest that there should be a common effect. This may be an effect on cell membranes. This includes fluidization of membranes and changes in composition of membrane phospholipids [350].

Chapter 19 Folate and anticonvulsant drugs

Evidence of folate deficiency is present among a significant number of patients treated with anticonvulsant drugs. Occasionally such patients develop a frank megaloblastic anaemia.

Anticonvulsant drugs The drug most commonly associated with the development of a megaloblastic anaemia is diphenylhydantoin (Phenytoin) but other drugs such as primidone (Mysoline), phenobarbital and other barbiturates have been implicated [7]. Effects on the blood and on folate metabolism have been demonstrated with carbamazepine and valproic acid. Many patients are treated with combinations of these drugs.

Haematology Macrocytosis has been reported in a significant proportion of treated epileptics ranging from almost zero to over half the

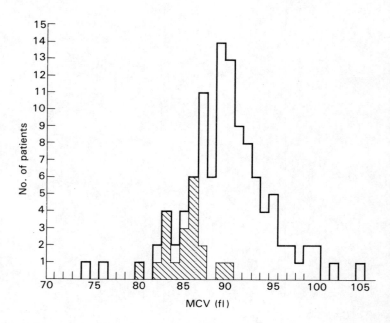

Fig. 19.1 The MCV was normal in 18 untreated epileptics ranging from 80 to 91 fl (hatched columns) and was increased in 42 out of 108 patients treated with diphenylhydantoin and primidone (open columns).

patients. Reynolds compared the MCV in 18 untreated epileptics with 108 treated patients. All the untreated patients had a normal MCV; the MCV was raised in 42 of the treated patients [7] (Fig. 19.1). Of the other hand others have failed to find any macrocytosis [351].

Three studies report on marrow changes in patients on anticonvulsant drugs. Megaloblastic changes were noted in 17 out of 45 patients in one study and in 49 out of 149 in a second [7]. A third study found megaloblastosis in 11 out of 14 patients including all the patients with a raised MCV [352]. The deoxyuridine suppression test was normal however in nine of these patients and abnormal in only two who had low red cell folate levels. The data suggest that macrocytosis and megaloblastosis may occur in anticonvulsant-treated patients as a result of the toxic effect of the drug (as with alcohol) and is generally not due to folate deficiency. Indeed the MCV was found not to fall on folate therapy [353].

Folate status The serum folate level was low in 52% of 1076 patients in 16 published series [7]. Serum folate levels tend to be lower in those taking more than one anticonvulsant drug.

Red cell folate levels too are low in about 10% of epileptics. In a recent study low red cell folate levels were present in 22% of patients taking several anticonvulsants, in 17% taking carbamazepine alone, in 13% taking phenytoin alone and in 9% taking sodium valproate alone [354]. Red cell folate levels tend to be lower in epileptics in institutions.

Formiminoglutamic acid excretion is generally normal or even low in patients on anticonvulsants. Possibly this is due to induction of enzymes that actively metabolize histidine and its products.

CSF folate levels are halved in treated epileptic patients, a mean of 11 ng folate/ml CSF as compared to 21 ng/ml in controls [7].

Cobalamin status The mean serum Cbl level is lower in anticonvulsant-treated patients. The mean serum Cbl level among 96 treated patients was 335 pmol/l as compared to 570 pmol/l in 727 controls [355]. Up to 6% of patients had low serum Cbl levels. Patients with megaloblastic anaemia due to anticonvulsants may have very low serum Cbl levels (down to 30 pg/ml) and these rise to normal on folate therapy alone. However, pernicious anaemia must not be overlooked in such patients. The cobalamin level in CSF has also been reported to be low — 9.7

pg/ml as compared to 17.8 pg/ml in controls [356]. Transient impairment of Cbl absorption may be present in patients with megaloblastic anaemia due to anticonvulsant drugs and disappears after folate therapy.

Pathogenesis of folate deficiency

The explanation for the development of folate deficiency in patients taking anticonvulsant drugs is not clear but may be a summation of a number of facets that each tend towards a negative folate balance.

The dietary folate intake among those on anticonvulsants was only two-thirds of that consumed by a control group [354]. Poor nutrition is a frequent factor in those developing a megaloblastic anaemia. Institutionalized patients tend to be most folate deficient probably for nutritional reasons.

Incubation of human marrow cells with diphenylhydantoin produces a dose-dependent impairment of DNA synthesis as assessed by impaired thymidine incorporation [357]. There is an impairment of proliferation of skeletal muscle cells by diphenylhydantoin *in vitro* [358] and of lymphocytes stimulated by phytohaemagglutinin [359]. The effect on lymphocytes *in vivo* may be the reason for reduced immunoglobulin levels in anticonvulsant-treated patients. Cells that are unable to complete DNA synthesis are phagocytosed and this leads to increased folate requirements.

There have been a number of attempts to assess intestinal absorption of folates when the oral folate was given with diphenylhydantoin. The studies were indecisive and failed to provide convincing evidence that anticonvulsants have an effect on gut function [7].

Another mechanism that may influence folate status by anticonvulsants is enzyme induction. Increased breakdown of labelled folate was demonstrated in mice given diphenylhydantoin but not when they were given phenobarbital [360]. In man diphenylhydantoin causes a fall in serum folate level [361] which was attributed to enzyme induction. On the other hand diphenylhydantoin has been reported to promote urinary excretion of newly absorbed folate given as pteroylglutamic acid and if this occurred with endogenous plasma methylH$_4$folate, it would be another explanation for the fall in serum folate [362]. Increased catabolism of endogenous folate in man, if it occurs, would lead to folate deficiency.

There is a one in ten risk that a pregnant woman on anticonvulsant drugs will produce a malformed child. The most frequent defects are cleft lip, skeletal anomalies, congenital heart disease, CNS defects, facial and ear abnormalities, mental retardation and genito-urinary defects. These problems appear to be overcome by giving folate (2.5–5 mg daily) from early pregnancy or even before conception [363]. Women giving birth to malformed infants had significantly lower blood folate levels than women who had a normal outcome [364]. Since congenital anomalies are prevented by folate, it strongly suggests that the drugs are influencing folate function directly.

The effect of anticonvulsants on folate coenzyme pathways have been explored by a few groups (Table 19.1). The changes observed in enzyme activity were not sufficiently consistent to indicate a clear pattern. A fall in folate polyglutamate level in rats following phenobarbital has been reported [369].

The peripheral neuropathy in man due to anticonvulsants is reversed by folates [6] again emphasizing the effect of the drug on folate metabolism. The mechanism remains to be elucidated.

Megaloblastic anaemia   Anticonvulsants can be associated with severe megaloblastic anaemia. In the case of diphenylhydantoin the average time on therapy before the diagnosis of megaloblastic anaemia is made is 6 years. About a quarter of patients are found to take an inadequate diet and multiple drug therapy is frequently

Table 19.1 Effect of anticonvulsant drugs on folates in the mouse [365] or rat [366–368]

	Diphenylhydantoin [365]	Primidone [366]	Valproate [367]	Phenobarbital [368]
Formate oxidation	↑	—	—	—
Histidine oxidation	↑	—	—	—
Methylene reductase*	↓	—	↓	↓ [†]
Methionine synthetase*	No change	No change	↓	No change
Serine hydroxymethylase*	—	↑	↑	No change
Methionine adenosyl transferase*	—	No change	↓	No change
S-adenosylmethyionine*	—	↑	↑	—
Folate*	No change	—	↓ [†]	↓
H₄PteGlu	↑	—	—	—
CH₃H₄PteGlu*	↓	—	—	—
Urinary folate excretion	No change	—	—	—

* In liver of mouse of rat.
[†] First few weeks of exposure only.
↑ increased; ↓ decreased.

present. A neuropathy resembling Cbl neuropathy has been described [7]. The anaemia is due to folate deficiency but almost half show a sub-optimal haematological response to Cbl therapy despite having normal Cbl absorption. Some patients have relapsed with recurring megaloblastic anaemia after cessation of folate therapy. In two out of 45 patients the anaemia was fatal [7].

Withdrawal of diphenylhydantoin in two cases and of primidone in one case was followed by a reticulocytosis although all three relapsed subsequently.

Folate therapy in some cases accelerates anticonvulsant drug metabolism and hence reduces the plasma levels of diphenylhydantoin and phenobarbital. Folate given 30 mg daily produced a significant shortening of the half-life of labelled diphenylhydantoin in chronic epileptics [370]. This may account for the increase in fit frequency reported in some studies [89,90].

In treatment of the megaloblastic anaemia the folate is given in the usual dose and no changes need be made in the medication required to manage seizures.

Variable consequences have been attributed to folate therapy in patients on anticonvulsant drugs. Folate in some studies increased the alertness of the patients, speed of thought and action, their confidence and sociability. Such improvements were apparent in 1–3 months of starting folate but in others took 6 months to appear. Others have failed to see any benefits from folate [7]. Withdrawal of a drug where possible has also improved clinical wellbeing. On the other hand in some, folate increased fit frequency and in several patients precipitated status epilepticus [89,90]. Other studies have not observed an effect on fit frequency.

Chapter 20　Chronic myelofibrosis and other myeloproliferative disorders

Severe folate deficiency leading to failure of haemopoiesis due to megaloblastic anaemia is relatively common in patients with chronic myelofibrosis. Clinically such patients may present as follows.

1 Megaloblastic anaemia in a patient with a very large spleen. The first diagnosis should be chronic myelofibrosis with folate deficiency.

2 Development of a transfusion requirement in a patient with chronic myelofibrosis. Although often this is due to marrow failure, not infrequently folate deficiency is the cause.

3 Development of thrombocytopenia in a patient with chronic myelofibrosis.

It is surprising how unaware clinicians are of the importance of folate deficiency in myelofibrosis and it only receives a bare mention in a monograph on myelofibrosis [371] and none in a recent review [372]. A definitive study of 49 patients was published in 1968 [273] although the first account of folate-responsive megaloblastic anaemia in myelofibrosis appeared 10 years earlier [373]. Other case reports have appeared since [374, 375]. Megaloblasts in myelofibrosis were first noted in 1923 [376].

Diagnosis　Diagnosis depends on demonstrating the presence of megaloblasts. This is complicated because failure to aspirate marrow (dry tap) is usual in myelofibrosis. However, it is also the rule that erythroblasts are normally present in peripheral blood in this condition and a buffy coat may show both megaloblasts and giant metamyelocytes. Occasionally some marrow can be aspirated and even when fragments are not forthcoming withdrawal of the marrow needle under strong suction with a 20 ml syringe often yields one or two drops of fluid that is rich in marrow cells. Of 49 patients seen over a 10-year period 16 were normoblastic, 16 at some stage had mild megaloblastic changes and 17 frank megaloblastic changes (Table 20.1).

161

Table 20.1 Comparison of 'mean' blood findings in patients with myelofibrosis who were normoblastic or megaloblastic [273]

Parameter	Normoblastic	Megaloblastic
RBC ($10^6/\mu$l)	3.5	2.9
Hb (g/dl)	10.8	8.7
PCV (%)	34	28
MCV (fl)	96	104
WBC ($10^3/\mu$l)	18	8
Platelets ($10^3/\mu$l)	272	130
Serum folate (ng/μl)	4.7	2.6
RBC/folate (ng/ml)	319	92
Serum Cbl (pg/ml)	963	1133

The range of serum folates in normoblastic patients was 3.0–6.6 ng/ml and in the megaloblastic group 0.7–6.0; red cell folates were 221–450 ng/ml in normoblastic patients and 48–133 in megaloblastic patients. In general 62% of all the patients with myelofibrosis in whom red cell folate levels were measured had abnormally low levels. The clearance from plasma of a small dose of folic acid was abnormally rapid in all 14 patients in whom it was performed [273]. With the exception of one patient who had associated pernicious anaemia, all had normal or more usually elevated serum Cbl levels.

Most patients with myelofibrosis not receiving folate prophylaxis will sooner or later show evidence of megaloblastosis due to folate deficiency. Folate prophylaxis, 5 mg two to three times weekly, is desirable.

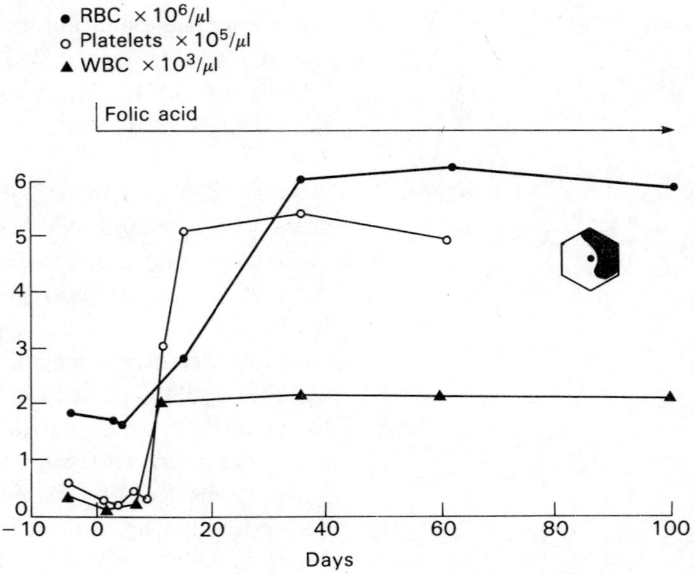

Fig. 20.1 Female, aged 62 years admitted to hospital with severe megaloblastic anaemia and massive splenomegaly. Folic acid 5 mg daily was followed by a reticuloscytosis of 22% and a rise in red cells, white cells and platelets. She had a raised serum Cbl level, a low red cell folate level and myelofibrosis was confirmed by marrow trephine biopsy.

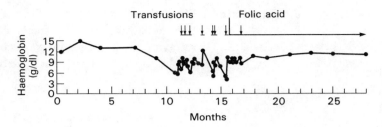

Fig. 20.2 Female, aged 57 years was known to have myelofibrosis of at least 8 years duration following polycythaemia. She had massive splenomegaly. A transfusion requirement developed and repeated transfusions over a year were given to maintain her haemoglobin level. Megaloblastosis was noted and folate therapy enabled her to maintain a haemoglobin level of 10 g/dl without further transfusions.

Response to therapy   Among 14 patients in whom frank megaloblastosis was noted, eight were described as having an excellent haematological response to folate, in two there was an increase in haemoglobin but in four folate did not have a significant effect. Some of these responses are illustrated in Figs 20.1 and 20.2. On occasion recognition of folate deficiency is life saving, for example, in patients with disappearing neutrophil or platelet counts. Folate has little effect when only minor megaloblastic changes are seen.

Cause of folate deficiency   There appears to be an abnormally high folate requirement in myelofibrosis, possibly due to increased marrow activity, the result of reduced red cell life span in this condition and ineffective haemopoiesis.

Polycythaemia rubra vera   Unlike myelofibrosis, patients with uncomplicated polycythaemia have normal serum and red cell folate levels [7].

Essential thrombocythaemia   These patients often have an abnormally rapid folate clearance suggesting that there is a high folate requirement.

Myelodysplastic syndrome   Over half the patients with sideroblastic anaemia were reported to have megaloblasts in marrow [377], although others have put the frequency at 20% [378]. Many of these show partial haematological responses to folate, although sideroblasts are unaltered. Sideroblasts and megaloblasts may also appear following treatment of tuberculosis with pyridoxine antagonists (cycloserine and pyrazinamide) and disappear on drug withdrawal.

Acute leukaemia   Megaloblasts in erythroleukaemia are unresponsive to folate therapy. More commonly megaloblasts are present in patients receiving folate antagonists such as methotrexate and anaemia due to methotrexate toxicity reversed by folinic acid is common.

Chapter 21   Chronic haemolytic states

Chronic haemolysis with a significant shortening of red cell life span and a hyperplastic marrow is associated with an increased folate requirement. Failure to meet this folate requirement from the diet can have devastating effects, particularly in children when additional requirements for growth and puberty are present. Not only is there megaloblastic haempoiesis which aggravates the severity of the haemolytic anaemia but there is delayed growth and puberty. While such problems may be rare in developed countries, they are relatively common among patients homozygous for haemoglobin S, patients with HbSC disease and HbS-thalassaemia in West Africa [379]. In Ibadan in one year 43 out of 405 new cases of sickle cell disease had megaloblastic anaemia. Had more marrow aspirates been done, many more would have come to light. Others had severe growth retardation and delayed puberty reversed dramatically by folate therapy, although the marrows were apparently normoblastic. These cases had haemoglobin levels below 6 g/dl and low platelet counts. Folate therapy was accompanied by a dramatic increase in growth and was followed by the onset of puberty. Four females over 20 years of age had never menstruated but following folate, regular menses were established.

Folate-deficient megaloblastic anaemia should be suspected when a patient with a chronic haemolytic state has a lower haemoglobin level than expected or has a reticulocyte count not consistent with the degree of haemolysis and haemoglobin level. The development of a transfusion requirement in a patient with chronic haemolysis who has previously maintained a steady haemoglobin level, should suggest folate deficiency [380]. Failure to respond to steroids, for example, in severe autoimmune haemolytic anaemia complicating chronic lymphatic leukaemia, can be due to megaloblastosis the result of folate deficiency. Pregnancy in patients with a chronic haemolytic state can precipitate megaloblastic anaemia due to folate deficiency and evidence for this emerges in the second trimester. In the absence of a haemolytic state megaloblastic anaemia in pregnancy is only manifest in the last weeks of pregnancy or in the puerperium. This has been described in relation to hereditary spherocytosis, ellipto-cytosis [7] as well as in sickle-cell syndromes.

Folate-deficient megaloblastic anaemia complicating severe thalassaemia syndromes has been described among others [7] in Arabs [380, 381] and Japanese [382]. The mean red cell folate among 76 controls was 436 ng/ml, among 55 patients with β-thalassaemia/Hb E disease it was 182 ng/ml and among 37 patients with Hb H disease it was 320 ng/ml [383]. About 30% of patients with thalassaemia/HbE and 4% of patients with HbH disease had red cell folates below the normal range. A low red cell folate is all the more significant in haemolytic states because young red cells normally have a higher folate content than older cells.

Megaloblastic anaemia in patients with sickle cell disease has been reported not only in Africa but in the USA [7] and elsewhere. Supplementation with folate in children with sickle cell disease in Jamaica resulted in a fall of the MCV by 4 fl as compared to a group receiving a placebo although there were no other differences between the groups [384].

The synthesis of HbS is depressed to a greater extent than HbA in folate deficiency. Indeed the level of HbS may decline to such an extent that the red cells no longer sickle under reducing conditions [385]. This is restored after folate therapy. Further, the amount of folate required to produce a response in megaloblastic anaemia with HbSS may be higher than in other patients. In one patient a supplement of 200 μg folate daily was without effect but 500 μg daily produced reticulo-cytosis [386]. In thalassaemia where the increased folate requirement is due to grossly ineffective haemopoiesis rather than extramedullary shortening of the red cell life span, folate therapy can be followed by very severe bone pain lasting for several days.

Megaloblastic haemopoiesis due to folate deficiency has been reported in paroxysmal nocturnal haemoglobinuria and haemolysis following Mycoplasma infection [7].

Confusion may sometimes arise because the direct anti-globulin test is positive in over one-third of patients with untreated pernicious anaemia as well as other megaloblastic anaemias [7]. It is probably due to adsorption of protein on the abnormal red cell surface and is usually due to complement. The reaction remains positive for 2–4 months. As mild jaundice and a raised bilirubin level occurs in untreated megaloblastic anaemia and as some response to steroid therapy occurs in pernicious anaemia, the possibility of serious diagnostic error exists for the unwary.

Prophylaxis with folate 5 mg on alternate days is desirable in patients with chronic haemolytic states, particularly where the diet is likely to be marginal in quality.

Chapter 22   Odds and ends

Acute pancytopenia

Acute 'marrow' failure can occur in very ill patients, often within the setting of an intensive care unit. In an analysis of 49 published cases, 37 (75%) had undergone major surgery, sepsis was present in 35 (71%) and 31 [65] were receiving total parenteral nutrition [387]. Thrombocytopenia with bleeding was a frequent feature.

Of 70 consecutive admissions to the intensive care unit of a single hospital, 22 patients had megaloblastic marrows. Eighteen of these 22 had received nitrous oxide anaesthesia during a major surgical procedure and 16 died. Only the patients receiving nitrous oxide had an abnormal dU suppression test indicating impaired Cbl–folate metabolism. Nitrous oxide inactivates Cbl and produces megaloblastosis in man. There were four megaloblastic marrows not associated with nitrous oxide. Two of these patients had acute alcohol intoxication, but the dU suppression in these and the other two patients were normal, indicating that the megaloblastosis was probably unrelated to Cbl–folate problems [388].

Apart from marrow failure, these patients have in common megaloblastic changes in marrow and a low serum folate. The data have been interpreted as folate deficiency of rapid onset in severely ill patients. It is difficult to conceive of a mechanism by which folate deficiency, other than due to the action of folate antagonists, can arise acutely. Megaloblasts can be a feature of dyshaemopoiesis, can be present as the result of drugs such as alcohol, diphenylhydantoin and others and can appear during the phase of recovery from marrow hypoplasia or marrow arrest. Some marrows in addition have ringed sideroblasts [389] a feature more common when there is toxic depression of haemopoiesis than in deficiency. The normal dU suppression in four such patients [388] implies that the appearance of megaloblasts in critically ill patients is not due to derangement of Cbl–folate pathways. A low serum folate is likely to be the result of the patients not eating subsequent to

168

the start of the illness or operation. Absorption of methyl folate from food is a major factor in maintaining serum folate levels. Folate therapy in these patients was probably started when the events leading to recovery had occurred including antibiotics, parenteral nutrition, etc. and it is difficult to ascribe recovery to folate treatment.

Others have attributed the changes seen in these patients to amino acid–ethanol mixtures given as parenteral nutrition [390] or to intravenous methionine [391]. A patient has been reported who developed gross megaloblastosis before death, had normal serum Cbl and serum folate levels and normal red cell folate levels (but 19 units of blood had been transfused) and an abnormal dU suppression (46%) corrected to 8% with folic acid. Possibly this patient was folate deficient before surgery [392].

Haemodialysis

Haemodialysis is accompanied by loss of folate into the haemodialysis fluid. Initial measurement indicated loss of 52 μg folate per dialysis [7] but subsequent data indicate a median loss of 37 μg which is equivalent to a loss of 16 μg daily if dialysis is done three times a week [393]. Red cell folates were normal in all but one out of 72 haemodialysis patients [393] but among 86 Danish patients eight had low red cell folate values [394]. In the last study 64 patients who were biopsied had normoblastic marrows. By contrast one of the early reports on this topic found that five out of ten patients were megaloblastic [395]. A higher proportion of patients have low serum folates — 14 out of 72 [393] — but serum Cbl levels are normal.

Although earlier views were that haemodialysis patients should receive a regular folate supplement, this has been questioned [393].

Exfoliative skin disorders

On occasion extensive long-term desquamation of skin appears to be the only explanation for megaloblastic anaemia due to folate deficiency. Hild first reported that two samples of normal skin had 0.5 and 1.4 μg folate/g and psoriatic skin 3.2–6.2 μg/g [396]. Others, however, have found a lower folate content 0.14 μg/g for normal skin squames and 0.32 μg/g for psoriatic squames [397], Even loss of 30 g of scales daily results in the loss of only 5 μg folate. Another study found that 50 g of squames was shed in psoriasis in 24 hours and their assays indicated a loss equivalent to 32 μg folate per day [398]. The latter is a much more significant loss and if continued for any length of time could indeed lead to folate deficiency if the dietary folate intake was marginal.

Although folate loss through desquamated nucleated skin squames is the most probable explanation for folate deficiency an additional mechanism has been postulated. Many patients with extensive psoriasis, erythroderma or eczema also have steatorrhoea which is alleviated when the skin disorder is brought under control [399]. The mechanism is not clear but Cbl and folate absorption are apparently unaffected and the biopsy appearance of the small gut remains normal. Nevertheless it does raise the possibility that impaired folate absorption is a factor in producing folate deficiency.

Methotrexate therapy of psoriasis can produce megaloblastic anaemia.

Neoplasia

The presence of megaloblasts on occasion in patients who have malignant disease was recognized at the turn of the century. If such patients have not received cytotoxic drugs and it is not due to associated pernicious anaemia then the likely cause is folate deficiency. Nevertheless folate deficiency is not common in such patients and the red cell folate was low in only one of 38 patients [400]. However, low serum folates, increased urinary formiminoglutamic acid excretion and an abnormally rapid clearance of an intravenous folate dose was present in 60–80% of patients, implying a negative folate balance [7]. Deprivation of folate for 5 months did not lead to any regression of tumour in seven patients [284]. Nor did folate therapy confer any benefit. An exception, however, is in patients with acute lymphoblastic leukaemia maintained on weekly methotrexate. In these subjects quite severe megaloblastic anaemia can result from overdosage and a short course of folinic acid is beneficial.

Oral contraceptives

If oral contraceptives have an effect on folate metabolism, then it is small. There were only minor differences in the mean MCV between 907 post-menopausal women (90.0 fl), 285 women taking oral contraceptives for 5 years (90.3) and 1746 menstruating women (88.9) [402]. Menstrual blood loss was about twice as great in the menstruating women as in those on the oral contraceptives implying that the lower MCV in the former relates to iron deficiency.

There are some 35 reports of women taking oral contraceptives who have had megaloblastic anaemia due to folate deficiency. Few have been investigated adequately but most of those who have, were found to have another factor contributing to folate deficiency such as coeliac disease or to have dietary deficiency. In a few patients reversal followed cessation of oral contraceptive usage [7]. The number of reports showing that the oral contraceptives caused a fall in serum folate or impaired folate absorption is equalled by the number of reports failing to show any effect [7].

Ten reports have found a lower red cell folate level in oral contraceptive users but three have not done so [403]. In one study the mean red cell folate value in oral contraceptive users was 261 ng/ml and non-users 293 ng/ml [403]. Women becoming pregnant within 6 months of stopping the contraceptive pill have lower red cell folate values (186 ng/ml) than controls (244 ng/ml) [404]. However, the frequency of iron deficiency in a group of women not taking oral contraceptives is higher than in a group taking oral contraceptives. About 15% of menstruating women have overt iron deficiency. The red cell folate per ng packed red cells is significantly higher in iron deficiency [405] and this is a possible explanation for differences in red cell folate levels between women taking oral contraceptives and others.

Thus minor differences in folate status are demonstrable in oral contraceptive users. It would be unwise to attribute the cause of megaloblastic anaemia to its use without rigid exclusion of other more significant factors. The effect, if any, of oral contraceptives on folate metabolism remains unproven.

Drugs   Folate antagonists that produce a megaloblastic anaemia are usually dihydrofolate reductase inhibitors [406, 407]. Methotrexate has been studied in greatest detail. Not only does it bind irreversibly to dihydrofolate reductase but it is a substrate to which pteroylpolyglutamate synthetase adds additional glutamic acid residues and *in vivo* methotrexate pentaglutamates have been identified. The methotrexate polyglutamates are probably able to compete with other folate polyglutamate coenzymes for aponezyme binding and so inhibit single-carbon unit transfers. Megaloblastic anaemia, sometimes fatal, has arisen from the use of methotrexate in the treatment of psoriasis. The effects of methotrexate as well as of other dihydrofolate reductase inhibitors, is reversed by supplying fully reduced folate such as formyltetrahydrofolate (folinic acid).

Other dihydrofolate reductase inhibitors have a much lower affinity for human dihydrofolate reductase while retaining a strong affinity for bacterial or plasmodial dihydrofolate reductase. Nevertheless when there is relative folate deficiency or poor renal function these compounds can cause megaloblastic anaemia in man which has proved fatal. In the United Kingdom 85 deaths associated with trimethoprim had been reported by 1985 of which 50 were due to blood dyscrasias. In these trimethoprim was given with sulphamethoxazole. Triamterene, a diuretic, has been associated with several examples of megaloblastic anaemia [7] and there is a report that it inhibits folic acid absorption [408].

Antimalarials are often dihydrofolate reductase inhibitors and these include pyrimethamine (contained in Fansidar and Maloprim) and Proguanil (Paludrine). Megaloblastic anaemia in malnourished Indian farm workers due to pyrimethamine [409] and due to Proguanil in patients with renal failure [410] have been reported.

Sulphasalazine is a drug widely used in the treatment of ulcerative colitis and more recently in rheumatoid arthritis. Most patients receiving more than 2.5 g daily have evidence of a haemolytic process due to direct damage to red blood cells. This includes abnormal red cell contraction, increased methaemoglobin levels, macrocytosis and reticulocytosis [411].

There are at least seven case reports of megaloblastic anaemia associated with sulphasalazine [412] and a report that two-thirds of patients taking the drug have megaloblastic marrow changes [413]. Megaloblastic anaemia was found in four out of 80 patients. These four had either coeliac disease, malnutrition or active red cell haemolysis and in three cases resolution of the anaemia and restoration of normoblastic haemopoiesis followed drug withdrawal [412].

Malabsorption of folate has been demonstrated in patients taking sulphasalazine by a number of methods. Recovery of unabsorbed [^{3}H]methyltetrahydrofolate in faeces after an oral dose of 3 µg/kg showed that absorption was impaired in all ten patients studied and recovered after drug withdrawal [412]. Using [^{3}H]pteroylglutamic acid and a urinary excretion method impaired folate absorption was present in untreated patients and was significantly worse after sulphasalazine, [414]. With a jejunal perfusion method impaired folate absorption and impaired hydrolysis of folatepolyglutamates in the gut in man was demonstrated in the presence of sulphasalazine [415].

In addition to an effect on folate absorption there are reports that sulphasalazine inhibits several enzymes in the rat concerned with folate metabolism *viz.* dihydrofolate reductase, methylenetetrahydrofolate reductase, serine transhydroxymethylase [416] and human intestinal brush border folate conjugase [417]. It was suggested that it interfered with a folate recognition site common to all these enzymes. Could the drug just be a cell toxic, action uncertain, having a similar effect on the gut and liver that it has on red blood cells and not necessarily having a specific effect on folate metabolism?

A fall in red cell folate levels has been demonstrated particularly in patients taking 2 g or more of sulphasalazine [418] and the level was low in nine out of 40 patients [413].

Megaloblastic changes occur after therapy with hydroxyurea, cytosine arabinoside, azathioprine. There are case reports suggesting that acyclovir, lithium, nitrofurantoin, arsenic, cyclophosphamide, tetracycline, vinblastine and even aspirin cause megaloblastic anaemia but further confirmatory reports are lacking.

Impaired Cbl absorption may occur in diabetic patients treated with oral hypoglycaemic agents of the biguanide group (phenformin, metformin and burformin). The serum Cbl level may be reduced. Cbl malabsorption may also occur with the administration of cholestyramine, colchicine, neomycin, para-aminosalicylic acid and even potassium supplements [7].

Acquired immune deficiency syndrome (AIDS)

No publication is complete without inclusion of the relation to AIDS. Fifteen to 36% of patients have been reported to have low serum Cbl levels and eight out of 11 apparently had impaired Cbl absorption [419]. No doubt the urine collections were complete. Zidovudine has been reported to reduce serum Cbl levels [420].

A syndrome resembling sub-acute combined degeneration of the cord has been described in an AIDS patient [421] and extremely low CSF folate levels have been reported in two children with neurological disease due to congenital infection with the AIDS virus [422].

Nitrous oxide and its abuse

N_2O inactivates Cbl [19] and hence methionine synthetase [82] of which Cbl is a co-enzyme. Inactivation of Cbl by N_2O is rapid, but recovery of methionine synthetase activity after withdrawal of N_2O is relatively slow requiring synthesis of new apoenzyme as well as a supply of new Cbl. In rats return of methionine synthetase activity after N_2O withdrawal takes 48–72 hours [82]. Thus inhalation of N_2O, even for very short periods, if repeated frequently, has a cumulative effect in potentiating Cbl inactivation. N_2O has been in use as an anaesthetic agent for more than 100 years. Its safety in a clinical context is unquestioned. However, there are special situations where N_2O exposure can lead to marrow failure or a neuropathy identical to that seen in PA.

Megaloblastic haemopoiesis can be demonstrated by marrow aspiration in some patients after *2 hours* N_2O exposure and the dU suppression test is abnormal [423]. This, however, is not manifest in routine blood counts, nor are the effects seen clinically. Cessation of N_2O inhalation sets in train the events that restore normality. Even *24 hours* of N_2O exposure is not accompanied by clinical problems although careful surveillance shows haematological changes [424, 425]. The marrow is then frankly megaloblastic with binucleate erythroblasts prominent [425]. Megaloblasts are still recognizable 3 days later and dyserythropoiesis follows. Giant metamyelocytes, abnormally large myelocytes and binucleate myelocytes appear early and persist for 5–6 days. Giant metamyelocytes become vacuolated. Hypersegmented neutrophils are first seen in the marrow after 5 days. The abnormal dU suppression becomes normal by day 7 after N_2O withdrawal.

The peripheral blood shows a fall in neutrophils from $8 \times 10^6/\mu l$ to $4 \times 10^6/\mu l$ by 2–4 days and hypersegmented neutrophils appear in the blood film on day 5, peak at day 7–9 and fall thereafter. The platelet count falls in the first 24 hours in all patients including controls not receiving N_2O.

N_2O inhalation persisting for *several days* was used to control spasms in patients with tetanus and led to pancytopenia, severe megaloblastc anaemia and, in some, death [20].

Intermittent exposure to N_2O may occur in those with access to the gas such as dentists and operating theatre personnel. Dentists may simply place the mask on their faces and inhale N_2O for 20–60 min or longer; others have inhaled from a surgical globe fitted with N_2O or use N_2O present in cartridges intended to prepare whipped cream [426]. Layzer [21] described 15 patients with prolonged N_2O exposure ranging from 3 months to several years. All but one were dentists and two were affected by inhaling N_2O in poorly ventilated surgeries. Symptoms included early sensory complaints such as numbness, tingling in hands or feet and loss of dexterity. Lhermitte's sign was present and there was loss of balance, leg weakness, gait ataxia, impotence and sphincter disturbances. Examination showed a polyneuropathy often with involvement of posterior and lateral columns of the spinal cord. CSF examination was normal. There were no abnormal blood findings and in three patients Cbl absorption remained normal. There were changes in nerve conduction. Improvement followed cessation of N_2O exposure, — in one patient within days but in others only after weeks or months. All the patients were able to work unassisted eventually, but in several moderate disability persisted. In some cases the neuropathy is accompanied by typical blood changes of a megaloblastic anaemia [427].

Another patient, using whipped cream cannisters as the source of N_2O, was confused and disorientated with periods of crying alternating with agitation. He exposed his genitalia, he was ataxic, and he showed memory loss, impaired concentration and recall. He recovered rapidly on N_2O withdrawal [429].

Occasionally intermittent N_2O exposure has been used to allow procedures that cause undue discomfort, for example daily physiotherapy in a patient with painful contractures. Thus N_2O/oxygen (1/1) given 3 times daily for 15–30 min each day caused megaloblastic anaemia after 24 days and again after 14 days [428].

A different situation is encountered when N_2O is given to patients with *undiagnosed subclinical Cbl deficiency*. Two such patients presented with subacute combined degeneration of the spinal cord 8 weeks after receiving an N_2O anaesthetic of 90 min duration [430].

Generally the serum Cbl level is normal but was low in 3 out of 10 patients abusing N_2O [430]. The onset of megaloblastic anaemia in those receiving prolonged N_2O can be prevented by large doses of formylH_4folate (30 mg folinic acid) [423, 431] given at the start of the procedure and repeated after 12 hours.

Although there have been suggestions that personnel exposed to trace amounts of N_2O in operating theatres or dental surgeries may suffer side effects and have an increased incidence of congenital malformation in offspring, these have not been substantiated.

Treatment is by withdrawal of N_2O. It is invariable that such patients also received Cbl but it is doubtful if Cbl hastens recovery.

References

1 Yusufji D, Mathan VI, Baker SJ. 1973. Iron, folate and vitamin B_{12} nutrition in pregnancy: study of 1000 women from Southern India. *Bulletin of the World Health Organization* **48**: 15–22.

2 Carmel R, Karnaze DS. 1986. Physician response to low serum cobalamin levels. *Archives of Internal Medicine* **146**: 1161–1165.

3 Hamilton HE, Ellis PP, Sheets RF. 1959. Visual impairment due to optic atrophy in pernicious anemia: report of a case and review of the literature. *Blood* **14**: 378–385.

4 Shorvon SD, Carney MWP, Chanarin I, Reynolds EH. 1980. The neuropsychiatry of megaloblastic anaemia. *British Medical Journal* **281**: 1036–1038.

5 Pincus JH, Reynolds EH, Glaser GH. 1972. Subacute combined degeneration with folate deficiency. *Journal of the American Medical Association* **221**: 496–497.

6 Figureroa AM, Johnson RH, Lambie DG, Shakir RA. 1980. The role of folate deficiency in the development of peripheral neuropathy caused by anticonvulsants. *Journal of the Neurological Sciences* **48**: 315–323.

7 Chanarin I. 1979. *The Megaloblastic Anaemias*. 2nd edn. Blackwell Scientific Publications, Oxford.

8 Heimburger DC, Krumdieck CL, Alexander CB, Birch R, Dill SR, Bailey WC. 1987. Localized folic acid deficiency and bronchial metaplasia in smokers: hypothesis and preliminary report. *Nutrition International* **3**: 54–60.

9 Killman S-A. 1964. Effect of deoxyuridine on incorporation of tritiated thymidine: difference between normoblasts and megaloblasts. *Acta Medica Scandinavica* **175**: 483–488.

10 Metz J, Kelly A, Swett VC, Waxman S, Herbert V. 1968. Deranged DNA synthesis by bone marrow from vitamin B_{12}-deficient humans. *British Journal of Haematology* **14**: 575–592.

11 Wickramasinghe SN, Matthews JH. 1988. Deoxyuridine suppression: biochemical basis and diagnostic application. *Blood Reviews* **2**: 168–177.

12 Hitzig WH, Kenny AB. 1975. The role of vitamin B_{12} and its transport globulins in the production of antibodies. *Clinical and Experimental Immunology* **20**: 105–111.

13 Bazzano G. 1969. Effects of folic acid metabolism on serum cholesterol levels. *Archives of Internal Medicine* **124**: 710–713.

14 Anderssen N. 1964. The activity of lactic dehydrogenase in megaloblastic anaemia. *Scandinavian Journal of Haematology* **1**: 212–219.

15 Hooton JWL, Hoffbrand AV. 1976. Thymidine kinase in megaloblastic anaemia. *British Journal of Haematology* **33**: 527–537.

16 Chanarin I, Malkowska V, O'Hea A-M, Rinsler MG, Price AB. 1985. Megaloblastic anaemia in a vegetarian Hindu community. *Lancet* **ii**:

1168–1172.

17 Hamilton HE, Sheets RF, DeGowin EL. 1958. Studies with inagglu-tinable erythrocyte counts. VII Further investigation of the hemolytic mechanism in untreated pernicious anemia and the demonstration of a hemolytic property in the plasma. *Journal of Laboratory and Clinical Medicine* **51**: 942–955.

18 Heath CW Jr. 1966. Cytogenetic observations in vitamin B_{12} and folate deficiency. *Blood* **27**: 800–815.

19 Zacharias W, O'Connor TR, Larson JE. 1988. Methylation of cytosine in the 5-position alters the structural and energetic properties of the supercoil-induced Z-helix of B-Z junctions. *Biochemistry* **27**: 2970–2978.

20 Banks RGS, Henderson RJ, Pratt JM. 1968. Reactions of gases in solution. Part III Some reactions of nitrous oxide with transition-metal complexes. *Journal of the Chemical Society*: 2886–2889.

21 Lassen HCA, Henriksen E, Neukirch F, Kristensen HS. 1956. Treat-ment of tetanus. Severe bone marrow depression after prolonged nitrous oxide anaesthesia. *Lancet* **i**: 527–530.

22 Layzer RB. 1978. Myeloneuropathy after prolonged exposure to nitrous oxide. *Lancet* **ii**: 1227–1230.

23 Stabler SP, Marcell PD, Podell ER, Allen RH, Savage DG, Linden-baum J. 1988. Elevation of total homocysteine in the serum of pa-tients with cobalamin or folate deficiency detected by capillary gas chromatography–mass spectrometry. *Journal of Clinical Investigation* **81**: 466–474.

24 Börgstrom B, Nordén Å, Åkesson B, Jägerstad M. 1975. A study of food. Consumption by the duplicate portion technique in a sample of the Dalby population. *Scandinavian Journal of Social Medicine* supple-ment **10**: 75–77.

25 Linnell JC, Hoffbrand AV, Hussein HAA, Wise IJ, Matthews DM. 1974. Tissue distribution of coenzyme and other forms of vitamin B_{12} in control subjects and patients with pernicious anaemia. *Clinical Science and Molecular Medicine* **46**: 163–172.

26 Ardeman S, Chanarin I, Doyle JC. 1964. Studies on the secretion of gastric intrinsic factor in man. *British Medical Journal* **ii**: 600–603.

27 Quadros EV, Rothenberg SP, Jaffe EA. 1989. Endothelial cells from human umbilical vein secrete functional transcobalamin II. *American Journal of Physiology* **256**: C296–C303.

28 Frater-Schröder M, Porak HJ, Erikssen AW, Daiger SP, Cavalli-Storza LL. 1982. Standardization of nomenclature of transcobalamin II variants. *Human Genetics* **61**: 165–166.

29 Sigal SH, Hall CA, Antel JP. 1987. Plasma R binder deficiency and neurologic disease. *New England Journal of Medicine* **317**: 1330–1332.

30 Levine JS, Allen RH, Alpers DH, Seetharem B. 1984. Immunocyto-chemical localization of the intrinsic factor–cobalamin receptor in dog ileum: distribution of intracellular receptor during cell matura-tion. *Journal of Cell Biology* **98**: 1111–1118.

31 Gräsbeck R, Kouvonen I. 1983. The intrinsic factor and its receptor — are all membrane transport systems related? *Trends in Biochemical Sciences* **8**: 203–205.

32 Chanarin I, Muir M, Hughes A, Hoffbrand AV. 1978. Evidence for intestinal origin of transcobalamin II during vitamin B_{12} absorption. *British Medical Journal* **i**: 1454–1455.

33 Heyssel RM, Bozian RC, Darby WJ, Bell MC. 1966. Vitamin B_{12} turnover in man. The assimilation of vitamin B_{12} from a natural foodstuff by man and estimates of daily dietary requirements. *American Journal of Clinical Nutrition* **18**: 176–184.

34 Doscherholman A, McMahon J, Ripley D. 1976. Inhibitory effect of eggs on vitamin B_{12} absorption: description of a simple ovalbumin ^{57}Co–vitamin B_{12} absorption test. *British Journal of Haematology* **33**: 261–272.

35 Chanarin I, Muir M. 1982. Demonstration of vitamin B_{12} analogues in human sera not detected by microbiological assay. *British Journal of Haematology* **51**: 171–173.

36 Whiteside MG, Mollin DL, Coghill NF, Williams AW, Anderson B. 1964. The absorption of radioactive vitamin B_{12} and the secretion of hydrochloric acid in patients with atrophic gastritis. *Gut* **5**: 385–399.

37 Siurala M, Lehtola J, Ihamäki T. 1974. Atrophic gastritis and its sequelae, results of 19–23 years follow-up examination. *Scandinavian Journal of Gastroenterology* **9**: 441–446.

38 Stabler SP, Marcell PD, Podell ER, Allen RH, Lindenbaum J. 1986. Assay of methylmalonic acid in the serum of patients with cobalamin deficiency using capillary gas chromatography–mass spectrometry. *Journal of Clinical Investigation* **77**: 1606–1612.

39 Chanarin I, England JM, Mollin C, Perry J. 1973. Methylmalonic acid excretion studies. *British Journal of Haematology* **25**: 45–53.

40 Briedis D, McIntyre PA, Judisch J, Wagner HN Jr. 1973. An evaluation of a dual-isotope method for the measurement of vitamin B_{12} absorption. *Journal of Nuclear Medicine* **14**: 135–141.

41 Brugge WR, Goff JS, Allen NC, Podell ER, Allen RH. 1980. Development of a dual label Schilling test based on the differential absorption of cobalamin bound to intrinsic factor and R protein. *Gastroenterology* **78**: 937–949.

42 Dawson DW, Sawers AH, Sharma RK. 1984. Malabsorption of protein bound vitamin B_{12}. *British Medical Journal* **288**: 675–678.

43 Jones BP, Broomhead AF, Kwan YL, Grace CS. 1987. Incidence and clinical significance of protein-bound vitamin B_{12}-malabsorption. *European Journal of Haematology* **38**: 131–136.

44 King EC, Leibach J, Toskes PP. 1979. Clinically significant vitamin B_{12} deficiency secondary to malabsorption of protein-bound vitamin B_{12}. *Digestive Diseases and Sciences* **24**: 397–402.

45 Chanarin I, James D. 1974. Humoral and cell-mediated intrinsic-factor antibody in pernicious anaemia. *Lancet* **i**: 1078–1080.

46 Rose MS, Chanarin I, Doniach D, Brostoff J, Ardeman S. 1974. Intrinsic-factor antibodies in the absence of pernicious anaemia. 3–7 year follow-up. *Lancet* **ii**: 9–12.

47 Chandler CJ, Wang TTY, Halsted CH. 1986. Pteroylpolyglutamate hydrolase from human jejunal brush borders. Purification and characterization. *Journal of Biological Chemistry* **261**: 928–933.

48 Cook JD, Cichowicz DJ, George S, Lawler A, Shane B. 1987. Mammalian folylpoly-γ-glutamate synthetase.4. *In vitro* and *in vivo* metabolism of folates and analogues and regulation of folate homeostasis. *Biochemistry* **26**: 530–539.

49 Kohashi M, Clement RP, Tse J, Piper WN. 1984. Rat hepatic uroprophyrinogen III co-synthase. Purification and evidence for a bound folate coenzyme participating in the biosynthesis of uropor-phyinogen III. *Biochemical Journal* **220**: 755–765.

50 Steenkamp DJ, Husain M. 1982. The effect of tetrahydrofolate on the reduction of electron transfer flavoproteins by sarcosine and dime-thylglycine dehydrogenases. *Biochemical Journal* **203**: 707–715.

51 Wagner C, Briggs WT, Cook RJ. 1984. Covalent binding of folic acid to dimethylglycine dehydrogenase. *Archives of Biochemistry and Biophysics* **233**: 457–461.

52 Tippett P, Danks DM. 1974. The clinical and biochemical findings in

three cases of hypersarcosinemia and one case of transient hypersarcosinuria associated with folic acid deficiency. *Helvetia Paediatrica Acta* **29**: 261–267.

53 Blom W, Fernandes J. 1979. Folic acid dependent hypersarcosinaemia. *Clinica Chimica Acta* **91**: 117–125.

54 Herman RH, Rosensweig NS. 1969. The initiation of protein synthesis. *American Journal of Clinical Nutrition* **22**: 806–812.

55 Hoppner K, Lampi B, Perrin DE. 1972. The free and total folate activity in foods available on the Canadian market. *Canadian Institute of Food Science and Technology Journal* **5**: 60–66.

56 United States Department of Agriculture. 1976. *Composition of Foods.* Agriculture Handbook No 8-1. Washington, US Department of Agriculture.

57 Paul AA, Southgate DAT. 1978. *The Composition of Foods*, eds McCance and Widdowson, 4th edn. London, HMSO.

58 Department of National Health and Welfare. 1977 *Canada Food Consumption Patterns Report.* Ottawa, DNHW.

59 Poh Tan S, Wenlock RW, Buss DH. 1984. Folic acid content of the diet in various types of British households. *Human Nutrition: Applied Nutrition* **38A**: 17–22.

60 Leslie GI, Rowe PB. 1972. Folate binding by the brush border membrane proteins of small intestinal epithelial cells. *Biochemistry* **11**: 1696–1703.

61 Perry J, Chanarin I. 1970. Intestinal absorption of reduced folate compounds in man. *British Journal of Haematology* **18**: 329–339.

62 Perry J, Chanarin I. 1973. Formylation of folate as a step in physiological folate absorption. *British Medical Journal* **ii**: 588–589.

63 Antony AC, Kane MA, Portillo RM, Elwood PC, Kolhouse JF. 1985. Studies of the role of a paticulate folate-binding protein in the uptake of 5-methyltetrahydrofolate by cultured human KB cells. *Journal of Biological Chemistry* **260**: 14911–14917.

64 Suleiman SA, Spector R. 1981. Purification and characterization of a folate binding protein from porcine choroid plexus. *Archives of Biochemistry and Biophysics* **208**: 87–94.

65 Wagner C. 1985. Folate-binding proteins. *Nutritional Reviews* **43**: 293–299.

66 Chanarin I, Perry J, Reynolds EH. 1974. Transport of 5-methyltetrahydrofolic acid into the cerebrospinal fluid in man. *Clinical Science and Molecular Medicine* **46**: 369–373.

67 Herbert V. 1962. Experimental nutritional folate deficiency in man. *Transactions of the Association of American Physicians* **75**: 307–320.

68 Skacel PO, Chanarin I. 1983. Impaired chemiluminescence and bacterial killing by neutrophils from patients with severe cobalamin deficiency. *British Journal of Haematology* **55**: 203–215.

69 Wilcken DEL, Dudman NPB, Tyrrell PA, Robertson MR. 1988. Folic acid lowers elevated plasma homocysteine in chronic renal insufficiency: possible implications for prevention of vascular disease. *Metabolism* **37**: 697–701.

70 Chanarin I, England JM. 1972. Toxicity of trimethoprim-sulphamethoxazole in patients with megaloblastic haemopoiesis. *British Medical Journal* **i**: 651–653.

71 Schwartz SO, Kaplan SR, Armstrong BE. 1950. The long term evaluation of folic acid in the treatment of pernicious anemia. *Journal of Laboratory and Clinical Medicine* **35**: 894–898.

72 Herbert V, Zalusky R. 1962. Interrelation of vitamin B_{12} and folic acid metabolism: folic acid clearance studies. *Journal of Clinical Investigation* **41**: 1263–1276.

73 Noronha JM, Silverman M. 1962. On folic acid, vitamin B_{12}, methionine and formiminoglutamic acid metabolism. In: *Vitamin B_{12} und Intrinsic Factor, 2,Europäisches Symposion*, ed. Heinrich HC, pp. 728–736. Stuttgart, Enke.

74 Lumb M, Chanarin I, Deacon R, Perry J. 1988. *In vivo* oxidation of the methyl group of hepatic 5-methyltetrahydrofolate. *Journal of Clinical Pathology* **41**: 1158–1162.

75 Lumb M, Chanarin I, Perry J, Deacon R. 1985. Turnover of the methyl moiety of 5-methyltetrahydropteroylglutamic acid in the cobalamin-inactivated rat. *Blood* **66**: 1171–1175.

76 Chanarin I, Deacon R, Lumb M, Muir M, Perry J. 1985. Cobalamin–folate interrelation: a critical review. *Blood* **66**: 479–489.

77 Stokstad ELR, Reisenauer A, Kusano G, Keating JN. 1988. Effect of high level of dietary folic acid on folate metabolism in vitamin B_{12} deficiency. *Archives of Biochemistry and Biophysics* **265**: 407–414.

78 Sourial NA, Brown L. 1983. Regulation of cobalamin and folate metabolism by methionine in human bone marrow cultures. *Scandinavian Journal of Haematology* **31**: 413–423.

79 Deacon R, Jennings P, Lumb M, Perry J, Purkiss P, Chanarin I. 1981. The effect of nitrous oxide-induced inactivation of cobalamin on plasma amino acids in the rat. *Scandinavian Journal of Haematology* **27**: 267–270.

80 Benevenga NJ, Radcliffe BC, Egan AR. 1983. Tissue metabolism of methionine in sheep. *Australian Journal of Biological Science* **36**: 475–485.

81 Das KC, Hoffbrand AV. 1970. Studies of folate uptake by phytohaemagglutinin-stimulated lymphocytes. *British Journal of Haematology* **19**: 203–221.

82 Tisman G, Herbert V. 1973. B_{12} dependence of cell uptake of serum folate: an explanation for high serum folate and cell folate depletion in B_{12} deficiency. *Blood* **41**: 465–469.

83 Deacon R, Lumb M, Perry J, Chanarin I, Minty B, Halsey M, Nunn J. 1980. Inactivation of methionine synthase by nitrous oxide. *European Journal of Biochemistry* **104**: 419–422.

84 Van der Westhuyzen J, Metz J. 1983. Tissue S-adenosylmethionine levels in fruit bats (*Rousettus aegypticus*) with nitrous oxide-induced neuropathy. *British Journal of Nutrition* **50**: 325–330.

85 Weir DG, Keating S, Molloy A, McPartlin J, Kennedy S, Blanchflower J, Kennedy DG, Rice D, Scott JM. 1988. Methylation defiency causes vitamin B_{12}-associated neuropathy in the pig. *Journal of Neurochemistry* **51**: 1949–1952.

86 Lawson DH, Murray RM, Parker JLW. 1972. Early mortality in the megaloblastic anaemias. *Quarterly Journal of Medicine* **41**: 1–14.

87 Tudhope GR, Swan HT, Spray GH. 1967. Patient variation in pernicious anaemia as shown in a clinical trial of cyanocobalamin, hydroxocobalamin and cyanocobalamin-zinc tannate. *British Journal of Haematology* **13**: 216–228.

88 Chisholm IA, Bronte-Stewart J, Foulds WS. 1967. Hydroxocobalamin versus cyanocobalamin in the treatment of tobacco amblyopia. *Lancet* **ii**: 450–451.

89 Chanarin I, Laidlaw J, Loughridge LW, Mollin DL. 1960. Megaloblastic anaemia due to phenobarbitone. The convulsant action of therapeutic doses of folic acid. *British Medical Journal* **i**: 1099–1102.

90 Reynolds EH, Chanarin I, Matthews DM. 1968. Neuropsychiatric aspects of anticonvulsant megaloblastic anaemia. *Lancet* **i**: 394–397.

91 Osler W, Gardner W. 1877. On the changes in marrow in progressive pernicious anaemia. *Canadian Medical and Surgical Journal* **5**: 385.

92 Scott E. 1960. The prevalence of pernicious anaemia in Great Britain. *Journal of the College of General Practitioners* **3**: 80–84.

93 Hippe E, Jensen KB. 1969. Hereditary factors in pernicious anaemia and their relation to serum-immunoglobulin levels and age at diagnosis. *Lancet* **ii**: 721–724.

94 Ardeman S, Chanarin I. 1965. Assay of gastric intrinsic factor in the diagnosis of Addisonian pernicious anaemia. *British Journal of Haematology* **11**: 305–314.

95 Laws JW, Pitman RG. 1960. The radiological features of pernicious anaemia. *British Journal of Radiology* **33**: 229–237.

96 Rode J, Dhillon AP, Papadaki L, Stockbrügger R, Thompson RJ, Moss E, Cotton PB. 1986. Pernicious anaemia and mucosal endocrine cell proliferation of the non-antral stomach. *Gut* **27**: 789–798.

97 Carney JA, Go VLW, Fairbanks VF, Moore SB, Alport EC, Nora FE. 1983. The syndrome of gastric argyrophil carcinoid tumors and nonantral gastric atrophy. *Annals of Internal Medicine* **99**: 761–766.

98 Borch K, Renvall H, Liedberg G. 1985. Gastric endocrine cell hyperplasia and carcinoid tumours in pernicious anaemia. *Gastroenterology* **88**: 638–648.

99 Sjöblom S-M, Sipponen P, Miettinen M, Karonen S-L, Järvinen HJ. 1988. Gastroscopic screening for gastric carcinoids and carcinoma in pernicious anemia. *Endoscopy* **20**: 52–56.

100 Zamcheck N, Grable E, Ley A, Norman L. 1955. Occurrence of gastric cancer among patients with pernicious anaemia at the Boston City Hospital. *New England Journal of Medicine* **252**: 1103–1110.

101 Borch K. 1986. Epidemiologic, clinicopathologic and economic aspects of gastroscopic screening of patients with pernicious anemia. *Scandinavian Journal of Gastroenterology* **21**: 21–30.

102 Varis K. 1983. Surveillance of pernicious anemia. In: *Precancerous Lesions of the Gastrointestinal Tract*, eds Sherlock P, Morson BC, Barbara L, Veronesi U, pp. 189–194. Raven Press, New York.

103 Tanaka N, Glass GBJ. 1970. Effect of prolonged administration of parietal cell antibodies from patients with atrophic gastritis and pernicious anemia on the parietal cell mass and hydrochloric acid output in rats. *Gastroenterology* **58**: 482–494.

104 Hillman RS, Adamson J, Burke E. 1968. Characteristics of vitamin B_{12} correction of the abnormal erythropoiesis of pernicious anemia. *Blood* **31**: 419–432.

105 Camilleri J-P, Bérault J, Picker M, Diebold J. 1973. Distribution des cellules immunosécrétrices dans la muqueuse gastrique humaine, a l'état normal et au cours des gatrites chroniques. A propos de 46 gastro-biopsies dirigées. *Biologie et Gastro-enterologie* **6**: 231–241.

106 Kaye MD, Whorwell PJ, Wright R. 1983. Gastric mucosal lymphocyte subpopulations in pernicious anaemia and in normal stomach. *Clinical Immunology and Immunopathology* **28**: 431–440.

107 Wodzinski MA, Forrest MJ, Barnett D, Lawrence ACK. 1985. Lymphocyte subpopulations in patients with hydroxocobalamin responsive megaloblastic anaemia. *Journal of Clinical Pathology* **38**: 582–584.

108 Ardeman S, Chanarin I. 1965. Steroids and Addisonian pernicious anemia. *New England Journal of Medicine* **273**: 1352–1358.

109 Mosbech J. 1953. *Heredity in Pernicious Anaemia. A proband study of the heredity and relationship to cancer of the stomach*. Munksgard, Copenhagen.

110 Eisenbarth GS, Wilson PW, Ward F, Buckley C, Lebovitz H. 1979. The polyglandular failure syndrome: disease inheritance, HLA type and immune function. *Annals of Internal Medicine* **91**: 528–533.

111 Ungar B, Mathews JD, Tait BD, Cowling DC. 1981. HLA-DR patterns in pernicious anaemia. *British Medical Journal* i: 768–770.

112 Van den Berg-Loonen EM, Hilterman TCM, Bins M, Nijnhuis LE, Engelfriet CP. 1982. Increased incidence of HLA-DR2 in patients with pernicious anemia. *Tissue Antigens* 19: 158–160.

113 Neufeld M, Maclaren NK, Blizzard RM. 1981. Two types of autoimmune Addison's disease associated with different polyglandular autoimmune (PGA) syndromes. *Medicine* 60: 355–362.

114 Eisenbarth G, Wilson P, Ward F, Lebovitz HE. 1978. HLA type and occurrence of disease in familial polyglandular failure. *New England Journal of Medicine* 298: 92–94.

115 Barkan AL, Kelch RP, Marshall JC. 1985. Isolated gonadotropic failure in the polyglandular autoimmune syndrome. *New England Journal of Medicine* 312: 1535–1540.

116 Wright PE, Sears DA. 1987. Hypogammaglobulinemia and pernicious anemia. *Southern Medical Journal* 80: 243–246.

117 Myers H, Bower BF, Hild DH. 1980. Pure red cell aplasia and the syndrome of multiple endocrine gland insufficiency. *American Journal of the Medical Sciences* 280: 29–34.

118 Beveridge BR, Bannerman RM, Evanson JM, Witts LJ. 1965. Hypochromic anaemia. A retrospective study and follow-up of 378 in-patients. *Quarterly Journal of Medicine, NS* 34: 145–161.

119 Joynson DHM, Jacobs A, Murray Walker D, Dolby AE. 1972. Defect of cell-mediated immunity in patients with iron-deficiency anaemia. *Lancet* ii: 1058–1059.

120 Atrah HI, Davidson RJL. 1988. Iron deficiency in pernicious anaemia: a neglected diagnosis. *Postgraduate Medical Journal* 64: 110–111.

121 Carmel R, Weiner JM, Johnson CS. 1987. Iron deficiency occurs frequently in patients with pernicious anemia. *Journal of the American Medical Association* 257: 1081–1083.

122 Cristallo M, Braga M, Agape D, Primiguani M, Zuliani W, Vecchi M, Sironi M, Di Carlo V, De Franchis R. 1986. Nutrional status, function of the small intestine and jejunal morphology after total gastrectomy for carcinoma of the stomach. *Surgery, Gynecology and Obstetrics* 163: 225–230.

123 Mellström D, Rundgren Å. 1982. Long-term effects after partial gastrectomy in elderly men. A longitudinal population study of men between 70 and 75 years of age. *Scandinavian Journal of Gastroenterology* 17: 433–439.

124 Pickford IR, Craven JL, Hall R, Thomas G, Stone WD. 1984. Endoscopic examination of the gastric remnant 31–39 years after subtotal gastrectomy for peptic ulcer. *Gut* 25: 393–397.

125 Turnbull AL. 1969. Comparison of the effects of vitamin B_{12} after partial gastrectomy. *Gut* 10: 659–661.

126 Lous P, Schwartz M. 1959. The absorption of vitamin B_{12} following partial gastrectomy. *Acta Medica Sccandinavica* 164: 407–417.

127 Fischer AB. 1986. The long term results following Billroth II resection for duodenal ulcer. *Laegeforeningens forlag*.

128 Flejou J-F, Owen ERTC, Smith AC, Price AB. 1988. Effect of vertical banded gastroplasty on the natural history of gastritis in patients with morbid obesity: a follow up study. *British Journal of Surgery* 75: 705–707.

129 Schilling RF, Gohdes PN, Hardie GH. 1984. Vitamin B_{12} deficiency after gastric bypass surgery for obesity. *Annals of Internal Medicine* 101: 501–502.

130 Halverson JD, Zuckerman GR, Koehler RE, Gentry K, Michael HE, DeSchryver-Kecskemeti K. 1981. Gastric bypass for morbid obesity: a

medical-surgical assessment. *Annals of Surgery* **194**: 152–160.

131 MacLean LD, Rhode BM, Shizgel HM. 1983. Nutrition following gastric operations for morbid obesity. *Annals of Surgery* **198**: 347–355.

132 Crowley LV, Olson RW. 1983. Megaloblastic anemia after gastric bypass for obesity. *American Journal of Gastroenterostomy* **78**: 406–410.

133 Stewart JS, Roberts PD, Hoffbrand AV. 1979. Response of dietary vitamin B_{12} deficiency to physiological oral doses of cyanocobalamin. *Lancet* **ii**: 542–545.

134 Britt RP, Harper CM, Spray GH. 1971. Megaloblastic anaemia among Indians in Britain. *Quarterly Journal of Medicine NS* **40**: 499–520.

135 Matthews JH, Wood JK. 1984. Megaloblastic anaemia in vegetarian Asians. *Clinical and Laboratory Haematology* **6**: 1–7.

136 Stene-Larsen G, Mosvold J, Ly B. 1988. Selective Vitamin B_{12} malabsorption in adult coeliac disease. *Scandinavian Journal of Gastroenterology* **23**: 1105–1108.

137 Dong A, Scott SC. 1982. Serum vitamin B_{12} levels and blood cell values in vegetarians. *Annals of Nutrition and Metabolism* **26**: 209–216.

138 Chanarin I, Stephenson E. 1988. Vegetarian diet and cobalamin deficiency: their association with tuberculosis. *Journal of Clinical Pathology* **41**: 759–762.

139 Abdulla M, Andersson I, Asp N-G, Berthelsen K, Birkhead D, Dencker I, Johansson C-G, Jägerstad M, Kolar K, Nair BM, Nilsson-Ehle P, Nordén Å, Rassner S, Åkesson B, Öckerman P-A: 1981. Nutrient intake and health status of vegans. Chemical analyses of diets using the duplicate portion sampling technique. *American Journal of Clinical Nutrition* **34**: 2464–2477.

140 Carmel R. 1978. Nutritional vitamin B_{12} deficiency. Possible contributory role of subtle vitamin B_{12} malabsorption. *Annals of Internal Medicine* **88**: 647–649.

141 Jadhav M, Webb JKG, Vaishaava S, Baker S. 1962. Vitamin B_{12} deficiency in Indian infants, a clinical syndrome. *Lancet* **ii**: 903–907.

142 Srikantia SG, Reddy V. 1967. Megaloblastic anaemia of infancy and vitamin B_{12}. *British Journal of Haematology* **13**: 949–953.

143 Zetterström R, Franzén S. 1954. Megaloblastic anemia in infancy. Megaloblastic anemia occurring in an infant of a mother suffering from pernicious anemia of pregnancy. *Acta Paediatrica* **43**: 379–385.

144 Lampkin BC, Saunders EF. 1969. Nutritional vitamin B_{12} deficiency in an infant. *Journal of Pediatrics* **75**: 1053–1055.

145 Higginbottom MC, Sweetman L, Nyhan WL. 1978. A syndrome of methylmalonic aciduria, homocystinuria, megaloblastic anemia and neurologic abnormalities in a vitamin B_{12}-deficient breast-fed infant of a strict vegetarian. *New England Journal of Medicine* **299**: 317–323.

146 Frader J, Reibman B, Turkewitz D. 1978. Vitamin B_{12} deficiency in strict vegetarians. *New England Journal of Medicine* **299**: 1319–1320.

147 Davis JR, Goldenring J, Lubin BH. 1981. Nutritional vitamin B_{12} deficiency in infants. *American Journal of Diseases of Children* **135**: 566–567.

148 Gambon RC, Lentze MJ, Rossi E. 1986. Megaloblastic anaemia in one of monozygous twins breast fed by their vegetarian mother. *European Journal of Pediatrics* **145**: 570–571.

149 Stollhoff K, Schulte FJ. 1987. Vitamin B_{12} and brain development. *European Journal of Pediatrics* **146**: 201–205.

150 Lampkin BC, Shore NA, Chadwick D. 1966. Megaloblastic anemia of infancy secondary to maternal pernicious anemia. *New England Journal of Medicine* **274**: 1168–1171.

151 Hoey H, Linnell JC, Oberholzer VG, Laurence BM. 1982. Vitamin B_{12} deficiency in a breast fed infant of a mother with pernicious anaemia.

Journal of the Royal Society of Medicine **75**: 656–658.

152 Johnson PR, Roloff JS. 1982. Vitamin B$_{12}$ deficiency in an infant strictly breast-fed by a mother with latent pernicious anemia. *Journal of Pediatrics* **100**: 917–919.

153 Danielsson L, Enocksson E, Hagenfeldt L, Rasmussen EB, Tillberg E. 1988. Failure to thrive due to subclinical maternal pernicious anemia. *Acta Paediatrica Scandinavica* **77**: 310–311.

154 Heaton D. 1979. Another case of megaloblastic anaemia of infancy due to maternal pernicious anemia. *New England Journal of Medicine* **300**: 202–203.

155 Isaacs PET, Kim YS. 1983. Blind loop syndrome and small bowel contamination. *Clinics in Gastroenterology* **12**: 395–414.

156 Brandt LJ, Bernstein LH, Wagle A. 1977. Production of vitamin B$_{12}$ analogues in patients with small bowel bacterial overgrowth. *Annals of Internal Medicine* **87**: 546–551.

157 Hoffbrand AV, Tabaqchali S, Mollin DL. 1966. High serum-folate levels in intestinal blind loop syndrome. *Lancet* i: 1339–1342.

158 Updegraff TA, Neufeld NJ. 1981. Protein, iron, and folate status of patients prior to and following surgery for morbid obesity. *Journal of the American Dietetic Association* **78**: 135–140.

159 Morris JA Jr, Selivanov V, Sheldon GF. 1983. Nutritional management of patients with malabsorption syndrome. *Clinics in Gastroenterology* **12**: 463–474.

160 Hocking MP, Duerson MC, O'Leary JP, Woodward ER. 1983. Jejunoileal bypass for morbid obesity. Late follow-up of 100 cases. *New England Journal of Medicine* **308**: 995–999.

161 Beró T, Pongrácz Gy, Jávor T. 1982. Vitamin B$_{12}$ malabsorption after jejuno-ileal bypass surgery. *Acta Medica Academiae Scientiarum Hungaricae* **39**: 79–84.

162 From H, Sarva RP, Ravitch MM, McJunkin B, Farivar S, Amin P. 1983. Effects of jejunoileal bypass on the enterohepatic circulation of bile acids, bacterial flora in the upper small inestine, and absorption of vitamin B$_{12}$. *Metabolism* **32**: 1133–1141.

163 Thompson WG, Wrathell E. 1977. The relation between ileal resection and vitamin B$_{12}$ absorption. *Canadian Journal of Surgery* **20**: 461–464.

164 Williams CN, Dickson RC. 1972. Cholestyramine and medium-chain triglyceride in prolonged management of patients subjected to ileal resection or bypass. *Canadian Medical Association Journal* **107**: 626–631.

165 Valman HB, Roberts PD. 1974. Vitamin B$_{12}$ absorption after resection of ileum in children. *Archives of Diseases of Childhood* **49**: 932–935.

166 McBrien MP. 1973. Vitamin B$_{12}$ malabsorption after cobalt teletherapy for carcinoma of the bladder. *British Medical Journal* i: 648–650.

167 Kinn A-C, Lantz B. 1984. Vitamin B$_{12}$ deficiency after irradiation for bladder carcinoma. *Journal of Urology* **131**: 888–890.

168 Ratzkowski E, Hochman A. 1968. Gastro-intestinal function after abdominal cobalt irradiation. *Acta Radiologica. Therapy Physics Biology* **7**: 417–432.

169 Duncan W, Leonard JC. 1965. The malabsorption syndrome following radiotherapy. *Quarterly Journal of Medicine NS* **34**: 319–329.

170 Anderson GC, Walton KR, Chanarin I. 1981. Megaloblastic anaemia after pelvic radiotherapy for carcinoma of the cervix. *Journal of Clinical Pathology* **34**: 151–152.

171 Baker SM, Bogoch A. 1973. Subacute combined degeneration of the spinal cord after ileal resection and folic acid administration in Crohn's disease. *Neurology* **23**: 40–41.

172 Best CN. 1959. Subacute combined degeneration of spinal cord after extensive resection of ileum in Crohn's disease. *British Medical Journal* **ii**: 862–864.

173 Harries AD, Heatly RV. 1983. Nutritional disturbances in Crohn's disease. *Postgraduate Medical Journal* **59**: 690–697.

174 Filipsson S, Hultén L, Lindstedt G. 1978. Malabsorption of fat and vitamin B$_{12}$ and after intestinal resection for Crohn's disease. *Scandinavian Journal of Gastroenterology* **13**: 529–536.

175 Beeken WL. 1975. Remediable defects in Crohn's disease. *Archives of Internal Medicine* **135**: 686–690.

176 Cooke WT, Swan CHJ. 1974. Diffuse jejuno-ileitis of Crohn's disease. *Quarterly Journal of Medicine NS* **43**: 583–601.

177 Kraus J, Schneider R. 1977. Pernicious anemia caused by Crohn's disease of the stomach. *American Journal of Gastroenterology* **71**: 202–205.

178 Friedman PA, Weinstein PP, Mueller JF, Allen RH. 1983. Characterization of cobalamin receptor sites in brush-border plasma membranes of the tape worm spirmetra mansoides. *Journal of Biological Chemistry* **258**: 4261–4265.

179 Ching HL. 1984. Fish tapeworm infections (diphyllobothiiasis) in Canada, particularly British Columbia. *Canadian Medical Association Journal* **130**: 1125–1127.

180 Donoso-Scroppo M, Rapsos L, Reyes H, Godorecci S, Castillo G. 1986. Anemia megaloblastica secundaria a infeccion por Diphyllobothrium latum. *Revista Médica de Chile (Santiago)* **114**: 1171–1174.

181 Nyberg W. 1960. The influence of Diphyllobothrium latum on the vitamin B$_{12}$-intrinsic factor complex. I. *In vivo* studies with Schilling technique. *Acta Medica Scandinavica* **167**: 185–187.

182 Von Bonsdorff B. 1977. *Diphyllobothriasis in Man.* Academic Press, London.

183 Hoffbrand AV. 1974. Anaemia in adult coeliac disease. *Clinics in Gastroenterology* **3**: 71–89.

184 Davidson LSP, Girdwood RH. 1948. The imbalance of vitamins with particular reference to folic acid. *Lancet* **i**: 360–363.

185 Weir DJ, Hourihane DO'B. 1974. Coeliac disease during the teenage period. The value of serial folate estimations. *Gut* **15**: 450–457.

186 Halsted CH, Reisenauer AM, Shane B, Tamura T. 1978. Availability of monoglutamyl and polyglutamyl folates in normal subjects and in patients with coeliac sprue. *Gut* **19**: 886–891.

187 Fry L, Seah PP. 1973. Criteria fot the diagnosis of dermatitis herpetiformis. *Clinics in Gastroenterology* **3**: 145–157.

188 Brow JR, Parker F, Weinstein WM, Rubin CE. 1971. The small intestinal mucosa in dermatitis herpetiformis. *Gastroenterology* **60**: 355–361.

189 Tomkins A. 1981. Tropical malabsorption: recent concepts in pathogenesis and nutritional significance. *Clinical Science* **60**: 131–137.

190 Cook GC. 1984. Aetiology and pathogenesis of postinfective malabsorption (tropical sprue). *Lancet* **i**: 721–723.

191 O'Brien W, England NWJ. 1971. *Tropical Sprue and Megaloblastic Anaemia.* Churchill Livingstone, London.

192 Tomkins AM, James WPT, Walters JH, Cole ACE. 1974. Malabsorption in overland travellers to India. *British Medical Journal* **3**: 380–384.

193 Baker SJ, Mathan VI. 1971. *Tropical Sprue and Megaloblastic Anaemia.* Churchill Livingstone, London.

194 Bayless TM, Wheby MS, Swanson VL. 1968. Tropical sprue in Puerto Rico. *American Journal of Clinical Nutrition* **21**: 1030–1041.

195 Thomas PK, Hoffbrand AV, Smith IS. 1982. Neurological involve-

ment in hereditary transcobalamin II deficiency. *Journal of Neurology, Neurosurgery and Psychiatry* **45**: 74–77.

196 Haurani FI, Hall CA, Rubin R. 1979. Megaloblastic anemia as a result of an abnormal transcobalamin II (Cardoza). *Journal of Clinical Investigation* **64**: 1253–1259.

197 Hall CA, Begley JA. 1982. Atypical cobalamin binding in the serum of congenital deficiency of transcobalamin II. *British Journal of Haematology* **51**: 65–71.

198 Fráter-Schröder M, Erton J, Steinmann B, Kierat L, Hitzig WH. 1982. Quantitative messung der neusynthese von trancobalamin II in der fibroblastenkultur-bedeutung in der diagnose des transcobalamin-II-mangels. *Schweizerische Medizische Wochenschrift* **112**: 1435–1436.

199 Hoffbrand AV, Tripp E, Jackson BFA, Luck WE. Frater-Schröder M. 1984. Hereditary abnormal transcobalamin II previously diagnosed as congenital dihydrofolate reductase deficiency. *New England Journal of Medicine* **310**: 789–790.

200 Frater-Schröder M, Hitzig WH, Sacher M. 1981. Inheritance of transocobalamin II (TCII) in two families with TCII deficiency and related immunodeficiency. *Journal of Inherited and Metabolic Disease* **4**: 165–166.

201 Rana SR, Colman N, Goh K–O, Herbert V, Klemperer MR. 1983. Transcobalamin II deficiency associated with unusual bone marrow findings and chromosomal abnormalities. *American Journal of Hematology* **14**: 89–96.

202 Burkart PT, Begley JA, Hall CA. 1984. Low serum cobalamin in disorders of cobalamin transport. *Blood* **64**: 1301.

203 Seligman PA, Steiner LL, Allen RH. 1980. Studies of a patient with megaloblastic anemia and an abnormal transcobalamin II. *New England Journal of Medicine* **303**: 1209–1212.

204 Carmel R, Ravindanath Y. 1984. Congenital transcobalamin II deficiency presenting atypically with a low serum cobalamin level: studies demonstrating the coexistence of a circulating transcobalamin I (R binder) complex. *Blood* **63**: 598–605.

205 Niebrugge DJ, Benjamin DR, Christie, D, Scott CR. 1982. Hereditary transcobalamin II deficiency presenting as red cell hypoplasia. *Journal of Pediatrics* **101**: 732–735.

206 Carmel R, Herbert V. 1969. Deficiency of vitamin B_{12}-binding alpha globulin in two brothers. *Blood* **33**: 1–12.

207 Luhby AL, Cooperman JM. 1967. Congenital megaloblastic anemia and progressive central nervous system degeneration: further clinical and physiological characterization and therapy of the syndrome due to an inborn error of folate transport. American Pediatric Society. 77th Annual meeting, p 48.

208 Lanzowsky P. 1970. Congenital malabsorption of folate. *American Journal of Medicine* **48**: 580–583.

209 Su PC. 1976. Congenital folate deficiency. *New England Journal of Medicine* **294**: 1128.

210 Santiago-Borrero PJ, Santini R, Perez-Santiago E, Maldonado N. 1973. Congenital isolated defect of folic acid absorption. *Journal of Pediatrics* **82**: 450–455.

211 Urbach J, Abrahamov A, Grossowicz N. 1987. Congenital isolated folic acid malabsorption. *Archives of Disease in Childhood* **62**: 78–80.

212 Ponez M, Colman N, Herbert V, Schwartz E, Cohen AR. 1981. Therapy of congenital folate malabsorption. *Journal of Pediatrics* **98**: 76–79.

213 Rosenblatt DS, 1986 Inborn errors of folate and cobalamin metabolism. In *Genetic Disorders and the Fetus*, ed Milunsky A. pp. 411–418. Plenum, New York.

214 Rosenblatt DS, Cooper BA. 1987. Inherited disorders of vitamin B_{12} metabolism. *Blood Reviews* **1**: 177–182.

215 Shinnar S, Singer HS. 1984. Cobalamin C mutation (methylmalonic aciduria and homocystinuria) in adolescence. *New England Journal of Medicine* **311**: 451–454.

216 Cooper BA, Rosenblatt DS. 1987. Inherited defects of vitamin B_{12} metabolism. *Annual Review of Nutrition* **7**: 291–320.

217 Ledley FD, Levy HL, Shih VE, Benjamin R, Mahoney MJ. 1984. Benign methylmalonic aciduria. *New England Journal of Medicine* **311**: 1015–1018.

218 Matsui SM, Mahoney MJ, Rosenberg LE. 1983. The natural history of the methylmalonic acidemias. *New England Journal of Medicine* **308**: 857–861.

219 Mahoney MJ, Hart AC, Steen V, Rosenberg LE. 1975. Methylmalonicacidemia: biochemical heterogeneity in defects of 5′-deoxyadenosylcobalamin synthesis. *Proceedings of the National Academy of Sciences, USA* **72**: 2799–2803.

220 Goodman SI, Moe PG, Hammond KB, Mudd SH, Uhlendorf BW. 1970. Homocystinuria with methylmalonic aciduria: two cases in a sibship. *Biochemical Medicine* **4**: 500–513.

221 Bartholomew DW, Batshaw ML, Allen RH, Roe CR, Rosenblatt D, Valle DL, Francomano CA. 1988. Therapeutic approaches to cobalamin-C methylmalonic acidemia and homocystinuria. *Journal of Pediatrics* **112**: 32–39.

222 Schuh S, Rosenblatt DS, Cooper BA, Schroeder ML, Bishop AJ, Seargeant LE, Haworth JC. 1984. Homocytinuria and megaloblastic anemia responsive to vitamin B_{12} therapy. An inborn error of metabolism due to a defect in cobalamin metabolism. *New England Journal of Medicine* **310**: 686–690.

223 Carmel R, Watkins D, Goodman SI, Rosenblatt DS. 1988. Hereditary defect of cobalamin metabolism (Cbl G mutation) presenting as a neurologic disorder in adulthood. *New England Journal of Medicine* **318**: 1738–1741.

224 Rosenblatt DS, Laframboise R, Pichette J, Langevin P, Cooper BA, Costa T. 1986. New disorder of vitamin B_{12} metabolism (Cobalamin F) presenting as methylmalonic aciduria. *Pediatrics* **78**: 51–54.

225 Huguley CM Jr, Bain JA, Rivers SL, Scoggins RB. 1959. Refractory megaloblastic anemia associated with excretion of orotic acid. *Blood* **14**: 615–634.

226 Tubergen DG, Krooth RS, Heyn RM. 1969. Hereditary orotic aciduria with normal growth and development. *American Journal of Diseases of Childhood* **118**: 864–870.

227 Smith LH Jr. 1973. Pyrimidine metabolism in man. *New England Journal of Medicine* **288**: 764–771.

228 Fox RM, O'Sullivan WJ, Firkin BG. 1969. Orotic aciduria. Differing enzyme patterns. *American Journal of Medicine* **47**: 332–336.

229 Rajantie J. 1981. Orotic aciduria in lysinuric protein intolerance: dependence on the urea cycle intermediates. *Pediatric Research* **15**: 115–119.

230 Fallon HJ, Smith LH Jr, Graham JB, Burnett CH. 1964. A genetic study of orotic aciduria. *New England Journal of Medicine* **270**: 878–881.

231 Van der Zee SPM, Lommen EJP, Trijbels JMF, Schretlen EDAM. 1970. The influence of adenine on the clinical feature and purine metabolism in the Lesch-Nyhan syndrome. *Acta Paediatrica Scandinavica* **59**: 259–264.

232 Rich KC, Arnold WJ, Palella T, Fox IH. 1979. Cellular immune deficiency with autoimmune hemolytic anemia in purine nucleoside

physphorylase deficiency. *American Journal of Medicine* **67**: 172–176.

233 Stoop JW, Zegers BJM, Hendrickx GFM, Siegenbeek van Heukelom LH, Stall GEJ, de Bree PK, Wadman SK, Ballieux RE. 1977. Purine nucleoside phosphorylase deficiency associated with selective cellular immunodeficiency. *New England Journal of Medicine* **296**: 651–655.

234 Heisel MA, Siegel SE, Falk RE, Siegel MM, Carmel R, Lechago J, Staff G, Nielsen PG, Cummings P. 1984. Congenital pernicious anemia: report of seven patients, with studies of the extended family. *Journal of Pediatrics* **105**: 564–568.

235 Levine JS, Allen RH. 1985. Intrinsic factor within parietal cells of patients with juvenile pernicious anemia. A retrospective immunohistochemical study. *Gastroenterology* **88**: 1132–1136.

236 Katz M, Lee SK, Cooper BA. 1972. Vitamin B_{12} malabsorption due to a biologically inert intrinsic factor. *New England Journal of Medicine* **287**: 425–429.

237 Yang Y-M, Ducos R, Rosenberg AJ, Catron PG, Levine JS, Podell ER, Allen RH. 1985. Cobalamin malabsorption in three siblings due to an abnormal intrinsic factor that is markedly susceptible to acid and protoelysis. *Journal of Clinical Investigation* **76**: 2057–2065.

238 Burman JF, Jenkins WJ, Walker-Smith JA, Philips AD, Sourial NA, Williams CB, Mollin DL. 1981. Absent ileal uptake of IF-bound vitamin B_{12} *in vivo* in the Imerslund-Gräsbeck syndrome (familial vitamin B_{12} malabsorption with proteinuria). *Gut* **26**: 311–314.

239 Rumpelt HJ, Michl W. 1979. Selective vitamin B_{12} malabsorption with proteinuria (Imerslund-Najman-Gräsbeck-syndrome): ultrastructural examinations on renal glomeruli. *Clinical Nephrology* **11**: 213–217.

240 Becroft DMO, Holland JT. 1966. Goat's milk and megaloblastic anaemia of infancy: a report of three cases and a survey of the folic acid activity of some New Zealand milks. *New Zealand Medical Journal* **65**: 303–307.

241 Rogers LE, Porter FS, Sidburg JB. 1969. Thiamine-responsive megaloblastic anemia. *Journal of Pediatrics* **74**: 494–504.

242 Viana MB, Carvalho RI. 1978. Thiamine-responsive megaloblastic anemia, sensorineural deafness, and diabetes mellitus: a new syndrome? *Journal of Pediatrics* **93**: 235–238.

243 Haworth C, Evans DI, Mitra J, Wickramasinghe SN. 1982. Thiamine responsive anaemia: a study of two further cases. *British Journal of Haematology* **50**: 549–561.

244 Mandel H, Berant M, Hazani A, Naveh Y. 1984. Thiamine-dependent beriberi in the "thiamine-responsive anemia syndrome". *New England Journal of Medicine* **311**: 836–838.

245 Abboud MR, Alexander D, Najjar SS. 1985. Diabetes mellitus, thiamine-dependent megaloblastic anemia, and sensorineural deafness associated with deficient α-ketoglutarate dehydrogenase activity. *Journal of Pediatrics* **107**: 537–541.

246 Branda RF, Moldow CF, MacArthur JR, Wintrobe MM, Anthony BK, Jacob HS. 1978. Folate-induced remission in aplastic anemia with familial defect of cellular folate uptake. *New England Journal of Medicine* **298**: 469–475.

247 Howe RB, Branda RF, Douglas SD, Brunning RD. 1979. Hereditary dyserythropoiesis with abnormal membrane folate transport. *Blood* **54**: 1080–1090.

248 Ek J. 1980. Plasma and red cell folate values in newborn infants and their mothers in relation to gestational age. *Journal of Pediatrics* **97**: 288–292.

249 Ek J, Behncke L, Halvorsen KS, Magnus E. 1984. Plasma and red cell folate values and folate requirements in formula-fed infants. *European Journal of Pediatrics* **142**: 78–82.

250 Roberts PM, Arrowsmith DE, Rau SM, Monk-Jones ME. 1969. Folate state of premature infants. *Archives of Diseases of Childhood* **44**: 637–642.

251 Bank MR, Kirksey A, West K, Giacoia G. 1985. Effect of storage time and temperature on folacin and vitamin C level in term and preterm human milk. *American Journal of Clinical Nutrition* **41**: 235–242.

252 Gray OP, Butler EB. 1965. Megaloblastic anaemia in premature infants. *Archives of Diseases of Childhood* **40**: 530–560.

253 Strelling MK, Blackledge GD, Goodall HB, Walker CHM. 1966. Megaloblastic anaemia and whole blood folate levels in premature infants. *Lancet* **i**: 898–900.

254 Boss GR, Erbe RW. 1981. Decreased rates of methionine synthesis by methylenetetrahydrofolate reductase-deficient fibroblasts and lymphoblasts. *Journal of Clinical Investigation* **67**: 1659–1664.

255 Freem JM, Finkelstein JD, Mudd SH. 1975. Folate-responsive homocystinuria and 'schizophrenia'. A defect in methylation due to deficient 5,10-methylenetetrahydrofolate reductase activity. *New England Journal of Medicine* **292**: 491–496.

256 Narisawa K. 1981. Folate metabolism in infantile type of 5,10 methylenetetrahydrofolate reductase deficiency. *Acta Paedatrica Japonica* **23**: 82–86.

257 Hyland K, Smith I, Bottiglieri T, Perry J, Wendel U, Clayton PT, Leonard JV. 1988. Demyelination and decreased S-adenosylmethionine in 5.10 methylenetetrahydrofolate reductase deficiency. *Neurology* **38**: 459–462.

258 Wendel, U, Claussen U, Diekmann E. 1983. Prenatal diagnosis for methylenetetrahydrofolate reductase deficiency. *Journal of Pediatrics* **102**: 938–940.

259 Shin YS, Pilz G, Endries W. 1986. Methylenetetrahydrofolate reductase and methyltetrahydrofolate methyltransferase in human fetal tissue and chorionic villi. *Journal of Inherited Metabolic Disease* **9**: 275–276.

260 Harpey J-P, Rosenblatt DS, Cooper BA, le Moël G, Roy C, Lafourcade J. 1981. Homocystinuria caused by 5,10-methylenetetrahydrofolate reductase deficiency: a case in an infant responding to methionine, folinic acid, pyridoxine and vitamin B_{12} therapy. *Journal of Pediatrics* **98**: 275–278.

261 Wendel U, Bremer HJ. 1984. Betaine in the treatment of homocystinuria due to 5,10-methylenetetrahydrofolate reductase deficiency. *European Journal of Pediatrics* **142**: 147–150.

262 Duran M, Ketting D, de Bree PK, van Sprang FJ, Wadman SK, Penders TJ, Wilms RHH. 1981. A case of formiminoglutamic aciduria. Clinical and biochemical studies. *European Journal of Pediatrics* **136**: 319–323.

263 Russell A, Statter M, Abzug S. 1977. Methionine-dependent formiminoglutamic acid transferase deficiency: human and experimental studies in its therapy. *Human Hereditary* **27**: 205–206.

264 Mudd SH, Ebert MH, Scriver CR. 1980. Labile methyl group balances in the human: the role of sarcosine. *Metabolism* **29**: 707–720.

265 Kwee HG, Bowman HS, Wells LW. 1985. A racial difference in serum vitamin B_{12} levels. *Journal of Nuclear Medicine* **26**: 790–792.

266 Jones PN, Mills EH, Capps RB. 1957. The effect of liver disease on serum vitamin B_{12} concentrations. *Journal of Laboratory and Clinical Medicine* **49**: 910–922.

267 Norredam K, Chainuvati T, Gimsing P, Hippe E, Viranuvatti V. 1983. Plasma cobalamin and transcobalamin in patients with primary carcinoma of the liver. A study from Thailand. *Scandinavian Journal of Gastroenterology* **18**: 229–232.

268 Paradinas FJ, Melia WM, Wilkinson ML, Portmann B, Johnson PJ, Murray-Lyon IM, Williams R. 1982. High serum vitamin B_{12} binding capacity as a marker of the fibramellar variant of hepatocellular carcinoma. *British Medical Journal* **285**: 840–842.

269 Burger RL, Waxman S, Gilbert HS, Mehlman CS, Allen RH. 1975. Isolation and characterization of a novel vitamin B_{12}-binding protein associated with hepatocellular carcinoma. *Journal of Clinical Investigation* **56**: 1262–1270.

270 Waxman S, Liu C-K, Shreiber C, Helson L. 1977. The clinical and physiological implication of hepatoma B_{12}-binding proteins. *Cancer Research* **37**: 1908–1914.

271 Jacob E, Herbert V, Burger RL, Allen RH. 1977. Atypical plasma factor associated with bronchogenic carcinoma and complexing with R-type vitamin B_{12}-binding proteins. *New England Journal of Medicine* **296**: 915–917.

272 Fischer E. 1972. Studies on the abnormal high binding capacity of blood for vitamin B_{12} in chronic myeloid leukemia. *Clinica Chimica Acta* **36**: 409–418.

273 Hoffbrand AV, Chanarin I, Kremenchuzky S, Szur L, Waters AL, Mollin DL. 1968. Megaloblastic anaemia in myelosclerosis. *Quarterly Journal of Medicine* **37**: 493–516.

274 Gilbert HS, Weinrab N. 1976. Increased circulating levels of transcobalamin II in Gauchers disease. *New England Journal of Medicine* **295**: 1096–1101.

275 Lindemans J, Abels J, Neijens HJ, Kerrebijn KF. 1984. Elevated serum vitamin B_{12} in cystic fibrosis. *Acta Paediatrica Scandinavica* **73**: 768–771.

276 Matthews DM, Beckett AG. 1962. Serum vitamin B_{12} in renal failure. *Journal of Clinical Pathology* **15**: 456–458.

277 Bates CJ, Fleming M, Paul AA, Black AE, Mandal AR. 1980. Folate status and its relation to vitamin C in healthy elderly men and women. *Age and Aging* **9**: 241–248.

278 Varadi S, Elwis A. 1964. Megaloblastic anaemia due to dietary deficiency. *Lancet* **i**: 1162.

279 Magnus EM, Bache-Wiig JE, Aanderson TR, Melbostad E. 1982. Folate and vitamin B_{12} (cobalamin) blood levels in elderly persons in geriatric homes. *Scandinavian Journal of Haematology* **28**: 360–366.

280 Elwood PL, Shinton NK, Wilson CID, Sweetman P, Frazer AC. 1971. Haemoglobin, vitamin B_{12} and folate levels in the elderly. *British Journal of Haematology* **21**: 557–563.

281 Infante-Rivard C, Krieger M, Gascon-Barré M, Rivard G-E. 1986. Folate deficiency among institutionalised elderly. Public health impact. *Journal of the American Geriatric Society* **34**: 211–214.

282 Rosenberg IH, Bowman BB, Cooper BA, Halsted CH, Lindenbaum J. 1982. Folate nutrition in the elderly. *American Journal of Clinical Nutrition* **36**: 1060–1066.

283 Jägerstad M, Nordén A, Åkesson B. 1979. Relation between dietary intake and parameters of health status. In: *Nutrition and Old Age*, eds Borgström B, Nordén A, Åkesson B, Adulla H, Jägerstad M, pp. 236–264. Universitets Forleget, Oslo.

284 Gailani SD, Carey RW, Holland JF, O'Malley JA. 1970. Studies of folate deficiency in patients with neoplastic diseases. *Cancer Research* **30**: 327–333.

285 Manzoor M, Runcie J. 1976. Folate-responsive neuropathy: a report

of ten cases. *British Medical Journal* i: 1176–1178.

286 Brocker P, Lebel C, Maurin H, Lods JC. 1986. Carences en folates chez les sujets âgés: intérêt de leur correction dans le traitement des troubles du comportement. *Seminar de Hôpital de Paris* **62**: 2135–2139.

287 Hercberg S, Chauliac M, Galán P, Devanlay M, Zohoun I, Agboton Y, Soustoe Y, Bories C, Christides J-P, Potier de Courcy G, Masse-raimbault A-M, Dupin H. 1986. Relationship between anaemia, iron and folacin deficiency, haemoglobinopathies and parasitic infection. *Human Nutrition* **40C**: 371–379.

288 Hercberg S, Galán P, Assami M, Assami S. 1988. Evaluation of the frequency of anaemia and iron-deficiency anaemia in a group of Algerian menstruating women by a mixed distribution analysis: contribution of folate deficiency and inflammatory processes in the determination of anaemia. *International Journal of Epidemiology* **17**: 136–141.

289 Areekul S. 1982. Folic acid deficiency in Thailand. *Journal of the Medical Association of Thailand* **65**: 1–4.

290 Klipstein FA, Rubio C, Montas S, Tomasini JT, Castillo RG. 1973. Nutrtional status and intestinal function among rural populations of the West Indies III Barrio Cabreto, Dominican Republic. *American Journal of Clinical Nutrition* **26**: 87–95.

291 Chase HP, Kumar V, Dodds JM, Sauberlich HE, Hunter RM, Burton RS, Spalding V. 1971. Nutrtional status of preschool Mexican-american migrant farm children. *American Journal of Diseases of Childhood* **122**: 316–324.

292 Bindra GS, Gibson RS, Berry M. 1987. Vitamin B_{12} and folate status of East indian immigrants living in Canada. *Nutrition Research* **7**: 365–374.

293 Goel KM, Logan RW, House F, Connell MD, Strevens E, Watson WH, Bulloch CB. 1978. The prevalence of haemoglobinopathies, nutritional iron and folate deficiencies in native and immigrant children in Glasgow. *Health Bulletin* **36**: 176–183.

294 Brown A. 1955. Megaloblastic anaemia associated with adult scurvy: report of a case which responded to synthetic ascorbate alone. *British Journal of Haematology* **1**: 345–351.

295 Jandl JH, Gabuzda GJ Jr. 1953. Potentiation of pteroylglutamic acid by ascorbic acid in anemia of scurvy. *Proceedings of the Society of Experimental Biology and Medicine* **84**: 452–455.

296 Zalusky R, Herbert V. 1961. Megaloblastic anemia in scurvy with response to 50 microgram of folic acid daily. *New England Journal of Medicine* **265**: 1033–1038.

297 May CD, Hamilton A, Stewart CT. 1952. Experimental megaloblastic anemia and scurvy in the monkey. IV. Vitamin B_{12} and folic acid compound in the diet, liver, urine and feces and effects of therapy. *Blood* **7**: 978–991.

298 Lewis CM, McGown EL, Rusnak MG, Sauberlich HE. 1982. Inter-actions between folate and ascorbic acid in the guinea pig. *Journal of Nutrtion* **112**: 673–680.

299 Herbert V, Jacob E, Wong K-TJ. 1977. Destruction of vitamin B_{12} by vitamin C. *American Journal of Clinical Nutrition* **30**: 299.

300 Newmark HL, Scheiner JM, Marcus M, Prabhudasai M. 1979. As-corbic acid and vitamin B_{12}. *Journal of the American Medical Association* **242**: 2319–2320.

301 Chanarin I, McFadyen I, Kyle R. 1977. The physiological macro-cytosis of pregnancy. *British Journal of Obstetrics and Gynaecology* **84**: 504–508.

302 Lewis D, Stockley RJ, Chanarin I. 1982. Changes in the mean cor-

puscular red cell volume in women with β-thalassaemia trait during pregnancy. *British Journal of Haematology* **50**: 423–425.

303 Ek. 1982. Plasma and red cell folate in mothers and infants in normal pregnancies. Relation to birth weight. *Acta Obstetsricaet Gynaecologica Scandinavica* **61**: 17–20.

304 Landon MJ, Hytten FE. 1971. The excretion of folate in pregnancy. *Journal of Obstetrics and Gynaecology* **78**: 769–775.

305 Herbert V, Colman N, Spivack M, Ocasio E, Ghanta V, Kimmel K, Brenner L, Freundlich J, Scott J. 1976. Folic acid deficiency in the United States: folate assays in a prenatal clinic. *American Journal of Obstetrics and Gynecology* **123**: 175–179.

306 Chanarin I, Rothman D, Ward A, Perry J. 1968. Folate status and requirement in pregnancy. *British Medical Journal* **ii**: 390–394.

307 Regina E, Giugliani J, Jorge SM, Goncalves AL. 1984. Folate and vitamin B_{12} deficiency among parturients from Porto Alegre, Brazil. *Revista de Investigation Clinica (Mexico city)* **36**: 133–136.

308 Fleming AF, Hendricks JD de V, Allan NC. 1968. The prevention of megaloblastic anemia in pregnancy in Nigeria. *Journal of Obstetrics and Gynaecology of the British Commonwealth* **75**: 425–432.

309 Hercberg S, Bichon L, Galan P, Christides J-P, Carroget C, Potier de Courcy G. 1987. Iron and folacin status of pregnant women: relationships with dietary intakes. *Nutrition Reports International* **35**: 915–930.

310 Zittoun J, Blot I, Hill C, Zittoun R, Papiernik E, Tchernia G. 1983. Iron supplements versus placebo during pregnancy: its effects on iron and folate status on mothers and newborns. *Annals of Nutrition and Metabolism* **27**: 320–327.

311 Rogozinski H, Ankers C, Lennon D, Wild J, Schorah C, Sheppard S, Smithells RW. 1983. Folate nutrition in early pregnancy. *Human Nutrition: Applied Nutrition* **37A**: 357–364.

312 Hercberg S, Galan P, Chauliac M, Masse-raimbault A-M, Devanlay M, Bileoma S, Alihonou E, Zohoun I, Christides J-P, Potier de Courcy G. 1987. Nutritional anaemia in pregnant Beninese women: consequences on the haematological profile of the newborn. *British Journal of Nutrition* **57**: 185–193.

313 Hall MH, Pirani BBK, Campbell D. 1976. The cause of the fall in serum folate in normal pregnancy. *British Journal of Obstetrics and Gynaecology* **83**: 132–136.

314 Giles C, Shuttleworth EM. 1958. Megaloblastic anaemia in pregnancy and the puerperium. **ii**: 1341–1347.

315 Chanarin I. 1985. Folates and cobalamin. *Clinics in Haematology* **14**: 629–641.

316 Chanarin I, Davey DA. 1964. Acute megaloblastic arrest of haemopoiesis in pregnancy. *British Journal of Haematology* **10**: 314–319.

317 Poelmann AM, Aanoudse JG. 1986. A pregnant woman with severe epistaxis — a rare manifestation of folic acid deficiency. *European Journal of Obstetrics and Gynecology and Reproductive Biology* **23**: 249–254.

318 Smithells RW, Sheppard S, Schorah CJ, Seller MJ, Nevin NC, Harris R, Read AP, Fielding DW. 1981. Apparent prevention of neural tube defects by periconceptional vitamin supplementation. *Archives of Disease in Childhood* **56**: 911–918.

319 Laurence KM, James N, Miller MH, Tennant GB, Campbell H. 1981. Double-blind randomised controlled trial of folate treatment before conception to prevent recurrence of neural-tube defects. *British Medical Journal* **282**: 1509–1511.

320 Baumslag N, Edelstein T, Metz J. 1970. Reduction of incidence of

prematurity by folic acid supplementation in pregnancy. *British Medical Journal* **i**: 16–17.

321 Tchernia B, Blot I, Rey A, Kalwasser JP, Zittoun J, Papiernik E. 1982. Maternal folate status, birthweight and gestational age. *Developmental Pharmacology and Therapeutics* **4** Suppl. 1: 58–65.

322 Iyengar L, Rajalakshmi K. 1975. Effect of folic acid supplement on birth weights of infants. *American Journal of Obstetrics and Gynecology* **122**: 332–336.

323 Prentice AM, Whitehead RG, Watkinson M, Lamb WM, Cole TJ. 1983. Prenatal dietary supplementation of African women and birth weight. *Lancet* **i**: 489–492.

324 Rolschay J, Date J, Kristoffersen K. 1979. Folic acid supplement and intrauterine growth. *Acta Obstetricaet Gynaecologica Scandinavica* **58**: 343–346.

325 Hansen H, Rybo G. 1967. Folic acid dosage in prophylactic treatment during pregnancy. *Acta Obstetricaet Gynaecologica Scandinavica* **46** Suppl. 7: 107–112.

326 Pippard M, Chanarin I. 1988. Iron and folate supplements in pregnancy. *British Medical Journal* **297**: 1611.

327 Metz J. 1970. Folate deficiency conditioned by lactation. *American Journal of Clinical Nutrition* **23**: 843–847.

328 Izak G, Rachmilewitz M, Zan S, Grossowicz N. 1963. The effect of small doses of folic acid in nutritional megaloblastic anemia. *American Journal of Clinical Nutrition* **13**: 369–377.

329 Meagher RC, Sieber F, Spivak JL. 1982. Suppression of hematopoietic-progenitor-cell proliferation by ethanol and acetaldehyde. *New England Journal of Medicine* **307**: 845–849.

330 Michot F, Gut J. 1987. Alcohol-induced bone marrow damage. A bone marrow study in alcohol-dependent individuals. *Acta Haematologica* **78**: 252–257.

331 Wu A, Chanarin I, Slavin G, Levi AJ. 1975. Folate deficiency in the alcoholic — its relationship to clinical and haematological abnormalities, liver disease and folate stores. *British Journal of Haematology* **29**: 469–478.

332 Savage D, Lindenbaum J. 1986. Anemia in alcoholics. *Medicine* **65**: 322–338.

333 Morgan MY, Camilo ME, Luck W, Sherlock S, Hoffbrand AV. 1981. macrocytosis in alcohol-related liver disease: its value for screening. *Clinical and Laboratory Haematology* **3**: 35–44.

334 Unger KW, Johnson D. 1974. Red blood cell mean corpuscular volume: a potential indicater of alcohol usage in a working population. *American Journal of Medical Sciences* **267**: 281–289.

335 Hines JD. 1969. Reversible megaloblastic and sideroblastic marrow abnormalities in alcoholic patients. *British Journal of Haematology* **16**: 87–101.

336 Cooper RA. 1980. Hemolytic syndrome and red cell membrane abnormalities in liver disease. *Seminars in Hematology* **17**: 103–112.

337 Sullivan LW, Herbert V. 1964. Suppression of hematopoiesis by ethanol. *Journal of Clinical Investigation* **43**: 2048–2062.

338 Wickramasinghe SN, Longland JE. 1974. Assessment of deoxyuridine suppression test in diagnosis of vitamin B_{12} or folate deficiency. *British Medical Journal* **iii**: 148–150.

339 Baker H, Frank O, DeAngelis B and the VA study group on alcoholic hepatitis. 1987. Plasma vitamin B_{12} titres as indicators of disease severity and mortality of patients with alcoholic hepatitis. *Alcohol and Alcoholism* **22**: 1–5.

340 Halsted CH. 1980. Folate deficiency in alcoholism. *American Journal of*

Clinical Nutrition **33**: 2736–2740.

341 Hunter CK, Treanor LL, Gray JP, Halter SA, Hoyumpa A Jr, Wilson FA. 1983. Effects of ethanol *in vitro* on rat intestinal brush-border membranes. *Biochimica et Biophysica Acta* **732**: 256–265.

342 Weir DG, McGing PG, Scott JM. 1985. Folate metabolism, the entero-hepatic circulation and alcohol. *Biochemical Pharmacology* **34**: 1–7.

343 McMartin KE, Collins TD, Bairnsfather L. 1986. Cumulative excess urinary excretion of folate in rats after repeated ethanol treatment. *Journal of Nutrition* **116**: 1316–1325.

344 Wilkinson JA, Shane B. 1982. Folate metabolism in the ethanol-fed rat. *Journal of Nutrition* **112**: 604–609.

345 Barak AJ, Beckenhauer HC, Tuma DJ, Badqkhsh S. 1987. Effects of prolonged ethanol feeding on methionine metabolism in rat liver. *Biochemical Cell Biology* **65**: 230–233.

346 Tamura T, Romero JJ, Watson JE, Gong EJ, Halsted CH. 1981. Hepatic folate metabolism in the chronic alcoholic monkey. *Journal of Laboratory and Clinical Medicine* **97**: 654–661.

347 Blocker DE, Thenen SW. 1987. Intestinal absorption, liver uptake, and excretion of ^{3}H-folic acid in folic acid-deficient, alcohol-consuming nonhuman primate. *American Journal of Clinical Nutrition* **46**: 503–510.

348 Charlton RW, Jacobs P, Seftel H, Bothwell TH. 1964. Effect of alcohol on iron absorption. *British Medical Journal* **ii**: 1427–1429.

349 Celada A, Rudolf H, Donath A. 1979. Effect of experimental chronic alcohol ingestion and folic acid deficiency on iron absorption. *Blood* **54**: 906–915.

350 Traschi TT, Rubin E. 1985. Biology of disease. Effects of ethanol on the chemical and structural properties of biologic membranes. *Laboratory Investigation* **52**: 120–131.

351 Rose M, Johnson I. 1978. Reinterpretation of the haematological effects of anticonvulsant treatment. *Lancet* **i**: 1349–1350.

352 Wickramasinghe SN, Williams G, Saunders J, Durston JHJ. 1975. Megaloblastic erythropoiesis and macrocytosis in patients on anti-convulsants. *British Medical Journal* **iv**: 136–137.

353 Jansen ON, Olesen OV. 1970. Subnormal serum folate due to anti-convulsive therapy. *Archives of Neurology* **22**: 181–182.

354 Goggin T, Gough H, Bissessar A, Crowley M, Baker M, Callaghan N. 1987. A comparative study of the relative effects of anticonvulsant drugs and dietary folate on the red cell folate status of patients with epilepsy. *Quarterly Journal of Medicine NS* **65**: 911–919.

355 Krause K-H, Berlit P, Bonjour J-P, Schmidt-Gayk H, Schellenberg B, Gillen J. 1982. Vitamin status in patients on chronic anticonvulsant therapy. *International Journal for Vitamin and Nutrition Research* **52**: 375–385.

356 Frenkel FP, McCall MS, Sheehan RG. 1973. Cerebrospinal fluid folate and vitamin B_{12} in anticonvulsant induced megaloblastosis. *Journal of Laboratory and Clinical Medicine* **81**: 105–115.

357 Reid C, Chanarin I. 1978. Effect of phenytoin on DNA synthesis by human bone marrow. *Scandinavian Journal of Haematology* **20**: 237–240.

358 Goyle S. 1983. Effect of phenytoin on proliferation and differentiation of mouse muscle cells *in vitro*. *Methods and Findings in Experimental and Clinical Pharmacology* **5**: 143–148.

359 MacKinney AA, Booker HE. 1972. Diphenylhydantoin effects on human lymphocytes *in vitro* and *in vivo*. *Archives of Internal Medicine* **129**: 988–992.

360 Kelly D, Weir D, Reed B, Scott J. 1979. Effect of anticonvulsant drugs on the rate of folate catabolism in mice. *Journal of Clinical Investigation* **64**: 1089–1096.

361 Richens A, Waters AH. 1971. Acute effect of phenytoin on serum folate concentration. *Proceedings of the British Pharmacology Society* **41**: 414–415.

362 Krumdieck CL, Fukushima K, Fukushima T, Shiota T, Butterworth CE Jr. 1978. A long-term study of the excretion of folate and pterins in a human subject after ingestion of ^{14}C folic acid, with observations on the effect of diphenylhydantoin administration. *American Journal of Clinical Nutrition* **31**: 88–93.

363 Biale Y, Lewenthal H. 1984. Effect of folic acid supplementation on congenital malformations due to anticonvulsive drug. *European Journal of Obstetrics, Gynecology and Reproductive Biology* **18**: 211–216.

364 Dansky LV, Andermann E, Rosenblatt D, Sherwin AL, Andermann F. 1987. Anticonvulsants, folate levels, and pregnancy outcome: a prospective study. *Annals of Neurology* **21**: 176–182.

365 Billings RE. 1984. Decreased hepatic 5,10-methylenetetrahydrofolate reductase activity in mice after chronic phenytoin treatment. *Molecular Pharmacology* **25**: 459–466.

366 Carl CF, Gill MW, Schatz RA. 1987. Effect of chronic primidone treatment on folate-dependent one-carbon metabolism in the rat. *Biochemical Pharmacology* **36**: 2139–2144.

367 Carl GF. 1986. Effect of chronic valproate treatment on folate-dependent methyl biosynthesis in the rat. *Neurochemical Research* **11**: 671–685.

368 Carl GF, Smith DB. 1984. Effect of chronic phenobarbital treatment on folates and one-carbon enzymes in the rat. *Biochemical Pharmacology* **33**: 3457–3463.

369 Formiggini G, Bovina C, Marchi-Marchetti M, Marchetti M. 1983. Pteroylpolyglutamates in liver of phenobarbitone-treated rats. *International Journal for Vitamin and Nutrition Research* **53**: 390–393.

370 Makki KA, Perucca E, Richens A. 1980. Metabolic effects of folic acid replacement therapy in folate-deficient epileptic patients. In: *Monitoring*, eds Johannessen SI, *et al.* pp. 391–398. Raven Press, New York.

371 Lewis SM. 1985. *Myelofibrosis. Pathophysiology and Clinical Management.* Marcel Dekker, New York.

372 Varki A, Lottenberg R, Griffith R, Reinhard E. 1983. The syndrome of idiopathic myelofibrosis. *Medicine* **62**: 353–371.

373 Chanarin I, Mollin DL, Anderson BB. 1958. Folic acid deficiency and megaloblastic anaemias. *Proceedings of the Royal Society of Medicine* **51**: 757–763.

374 Hooey MA, Crookston JH, Squires AH. 1965. Myeloproliferative disease complicated by megaloblastic anemia and hyperuricemia. *Canadian Medical Association Journal* **93**: 935–937.

375 Tobin MS, Kim K-S. 1972. Reversibility in agnogenic myeloid metaplasia. *New York State Journal of Medicine* **72**: 3001–3004.

376 Minot GR, Buckman TE. 1923. Erythemia (polycythemia rubra vera). *American Journal of Medical Sciences* **166**: 469.

377 MacGibbon BH, Mollin DL. 1965. Sideroblastic anaemia in man: observations on seventy cases. *British Journal of Haematology* **11**: 59–69.

378 Kushner JP, Lee GR, Wintrobe MM, Cartwright GE. 1971. Idiopathic refractory sideroblastic anaemia. Clinical and laboratory investigation of 17 patients and review of the literature. *Medicine* **50**: 139–159.

379 Watson-Williams EJ. 1962. Folic acid deficiency in sickle-cell anaemia. *East African Medical Journal* **39**: 213–221.

380 Chanarin I, Dacie JV, Mollin DL. 1959. Folic acid deficiency in haemolytic anaemia. *British Journal of Haematology* **5**: 245–256.

381 Danel P, Girat R, Tchernia G. 1983. Thalassémie majeure révélée par une anémie mégaloblastique par déficit en folates. *Archives Francais*

Pediatrique **40**: 799–801.

382 Imamura T, Yokota E, Naito Y, Kagimoto M, Naritomi Y, Kawaguchi T, Sugihara J, Ohta Y. 1985. Thalassaemia in Japan. *Acta Haematologica Japan* **48**: 2029–2037.

383 Vatanavicharn S, Anuvatanakulchai M, Na-Nakorn S, Wasi P. 1979. Serum erythrocyte folate levels in thalassaemic patients in Thailand. *Scandinavian Journal of Haematology* **22**: 241–245.

384 Rabb LM, Grandison Y, Mason K, Hayes RJ, Serjeant B, Serjeant GR. 1983. A trial of folate supplementation in children with homozygous sickle cell disease. *British Journal of Haematology* **54**: 589–594.

385 Heller P, Yakulis VJ, Epstein RB, Friedland S. 1963. Variation in the amount of hemoglobin S in a patient with sickle cell trait and megaloblastic anemia. *Blood* **21**: 499–483.

386 Alperin JB. 1967. Folic acid deficiency complicating sickle cell anemia. *Archives of Internal Medicine* **120**: 298–306.

387 Lawlor E, Watson E, Keogh JAB. 1983. Folate deficiency in acutely ill patients. *Irish Journal of Medical Science* **152**: 73–82.

388 Amos RJ, Amess JAL, Hinds CJ, Mollin DL. 1982. Incidence and pathogenesis of acute megaloblastic bone-marrow change in patients reseiving intensive care. *Lancet* **ii**: 835–839.

389 Densburg J, Bensen W, Ali MAM, McBride J, Ciok J. 1977. Megaloblastic anemia in patients receiving total parenteral nutrition without folic acid or vitamin B_{12} supplementation. *Canadian Medical Journal* **117**: 144–146.

390 Wardrop CAJ, Heatley RV, Tennant GB, Hughes LE. 1975. Acute folate deficiency in surgical patients on aminoacid/ethanol intravenous nutrition. *Lancet* **ii**: 640–642.

391 Connor H, Newton DJ, Preston FE, Woods HF. 1978. Oral methionine loading as a cause of acute serum folate deficiency: its relevance to parenteral nutrition. *Postgraduate Medical Journal* **54**: 318–320.

392 Beard MEJ, Hatipov CS, Hamer JW. 1978. Acute marrow folate deficiency during intensive care. *British Medical Journal* **i**: 624–625.

393 Cunningham J, Sharman VL, Goodwin FJ, Marsh FP. 1981. Do patients receiving haemodialysis need folic acid supplements. *British Medical Journal* **ii**: 1582.

394 Milman N. 1980. Serum vitamin B_{12} and erythrocyte folate in chronic uraemia and after renal transplantation. *Scandinavian Journal of Haematology* **25**: 151–157.

395 Hampers CL, Streiff R, Nathan DC, Snyder D, Merrill JP. 1967. Megaloblastic hematopoiesis in uremia and in patients on long term hemodialysis. *New England Journal of Medicine* **276**: 551–554.

396 Hild DE. 1969. Folate losses from the skin in exfoliative dermatitis. *Archives of Internal Medicine* **123**: 51–54.

397 Fry L, MacDonald A, Almeyda J, Griffin CJ, Hoffbrand AV. 1971. The mechanism of folate deficiency in psoriasis. *British Journal of Dermatology* **84**: 539–544.

398 Touraine R, Revuz J, Zittoun J, Jarret J, Tulliez M. 1973. Study of folate in psoriasis: blood levels, intestinal absorption and cutaneous loss. *British Journal of Dermatology* **89**: 335–341.

399 Shuster S, Marks J, Chanarin I. 1967. Folic acid deficiency in patients with skin disease. *British Journal of Dermatology* **79**: 398–402.

400 Magnus EM. 1967. Folate activity in serum and red cells of patients with cancer. *Cancer Research* **27**: 490–497.

401 Chick J. 1982. Epidemiology of alcohol use and its hazards with a note on screening methods. *British Medical Bulletin* **38**: 3–8.

402 Fisch IR, Freedman, SH. 1973. Oral contraceptives and the red blood cell. *Clinical Pharmacology and Therapeutics* **14**: 245–249.

403 Shojania AM. 1982. Oral contraceptives: effects on folate and vitamin B_{12} metabolism. *Canadian Medical Association Journal* **126**: 244–247.

404 Martinez O, Roe DA. 1977. Effect of oral contraceptives on blood folate levels in pregnancy. *American Journal of Obstetrics and Gynecology* **128**: 255–261.

405 Omer A, Finlaysen NDC, Shearman DJC, Samson RR, Girdwood RH. 1970. Plasma and erythrocyte folate in iron deficiency and folate deficiency. *Blood* **35**: 821–828.

406 Scott JM, Weir DG. 1980. Drug-induced megaloblastic change. *Clinics in Haematology* **9**: 587–606.

407 Lambie DG, Johnson RH. 1985. Drugs and folate metabolism. *Drugs* **30**: 145–155.

408 Zimmerman J, Selhub J, Rosensberg H. 1986. Competitive inhibition of folic acid absorption in rat jejunum by triamterene. *Journal of Laboratory and Clinical Medicine* **108**: 272–276.

409 Laing SRS. 1957. Refractory anaemia, a problem in diagnosis and epedemiology in a tea garden in Assam. *Journal of Tropical Medicine and hygiene* **60**: 131–136.

410 Boots M, Phillips M, Curtis JR. 1982. Megaloblastic anemia and pancytopenia due to proguanil in patients with chronic renal failure. *Clinical Nephrology* **18**: 106–108.

411 Pounder RE, Craven ER, Henthorn JS, Bannatyne JM. 1975. Red cell abnormalities associated with sulphasalazine maintenence therapy for ulcerative colitis. *Gut* **16**: 181–185.

412 Swinson CM, Parry J, Lumb M, Levi AJ. 1981. Role of sulphasalazine in the aetiology of folate deficiency in ulcerative colitis. *Gut* **22**: 456–461.

413 Elsborg L, Larsen L. 1979. Folate deficiency in chronic inflammatory bowel diseases. *Scandinavian Journal of Gastroenterology* **14**: 1019–1024.

414 Franklin JL, Rosenberg IH. 1973. Impaired folic acid absorption in inflammatory bowel disease: effects of salicylazosulfapyridine (azulfidine). *Gastroenterology* **64**: 517–525.

415 Halsted CH, Gandhi G, Tamura T. 1981. Sulfasalazine inhibits the absorption of folates in ulcerative colitis. *New England Journal of Medicine* **305**: 1513–1517.

416 Selhub J, Dhar GJ, Rosenberg IH. 1978. Inhibition of folate enzymes by sulfasalazine. *Journal of Clinical Investigation* **61**: 221–224.

417 Reisenauer AM, Halsted CH. 1981. Human jejunal brush border folate conjugase. Characteristics and inhibition by salicylazasulfapyridine *Biochimica et Biophysica Acta* **659**: 62–69.

418 Longstreth GF, Green R. 1983. Folate status in patients receiving maintenance doses of sulfasalazine. *Archives of Internal Medicine* **143**: 902–904.

419 Herbert V. 1988. B_{12} deficiency in AIDS. *Journal of the American Medical Association* **260**: 2837.

420 Richmond DD, Fischl MA, Grieca MH. 1987. The toxicity of AZT in the treatment of patients with AIDS and AIDS-related complex. *New England Journal of Medicine* **317**: 192–198.

421 Petito CK, Navia BA, Cho E-S, Jordan BD, George DC, Price RW. 1985. Vacuolar myelopathy pathologically resembling subacute combined degeneration in patients with the acquired immune deficiency syndrome. *New England Journal of Medicine* **312**: 875–879.

422 Smith I, Howells DW, Kendel B, Levinsky R, Hyland K. 1987. Folate deficiency and demyelination in AIDS. *Lancet* **ii**: 215.

423 Nunn JF, Chanarin I, Tanner AG, Owen ERTC. 1986. Megaloblastic bone marrow changes after repeated nitrous oxide anaesthesia. Reversal with folinic acid. *British Journal of Anaesthesis* **58**: 1469–1470.

424 Amess JAL, Burman JF, Rees GM, Nancekievill DG, Mollin DL. 1978. Megaloblastic haemopoiesis in patients receiving nitrous oxide. *Lancet* **2**: 339–342.

425 Skacel PD, Hewlett AM, Lewis JD, Lumb M, Nunn JF, Chanarin I. 1983. Studies on the haemopoietic toxicity of nitrous oxide in man. *British Journal of Haematology* **53**: 189–200.

426 Sahenk Z, Mendell JR, Couri D, Nachtman J. 1978. Polyneuropathy from inhalation of N_2O cartridges through a whipped-cream dispenser. *Neurology* **28**: 485–487.

427 Blanco G, Peters HA. 1983. Myeloneuropathy and macrocytosis associated with nitrous oxide abuse. *Archives of Neurology* **40**: 416–418.

428 Nunn JF, Sharer NM, Gorchein A, Jones JA: Wickramasinghe SN. 1982. Megaloblastic haemopoiesis after multiple short-term exposure to nitrous oxide. *Lancet* **i**: 1379–1381.

429 Sterman AB, Coyle PK. 1983. Subacute toxic delirium following nitrous oxide abuse. *Archives of Neurology* **40**: 446–447.

430 Schilling RF. 1986. Is nitrous oxide a dangerous anaesthetic for vitamin B_{12}-deficient subjects? *Journal of the American Medical Association* **255**: 1605–1606.

431 Amos RJ, Amess JAL, Nancekievill DG, Rees GM. 1984. Prevention of nitrous oxide-induced megaloblastic changes in bone marrow using folinic acid. *British Journal of Anaesthesia* **56**: 103–107.

432 Dawson DW, Lewis MJ, Wadsworth L. 1975. Changes in erythroblast morphology as an index of response to cyanocobalamin in patients with megaloblastic anaemic. *British Journal of Haematology* **31**: 77–85.

433 Brady T, Watson JE, Stokstad ELR. 1982. Folate pentaglutamate and folate hexaglutamate mediated one-carbon metabolism. *Biochemistry* **21**: 276–282.

434 Doerfler W. 1983. DNA methylation and gene activity. *Annual Review of Biochemistry* **52**: 93–124.

435 Zachau-Christiasen B, Hoff-Jørgenson E. Østergård-Kristensen HP. 1962. The relative haemoglobin, iron, vitamin B_{12} and folic acid values in the blood of mothers and their newborn infants. *Danish Medical Bulletin* **9**: 157–166.

436 Perry TL, Applegarth DA, Evans ME, Hansen S. 1975. Metabolic studies of a family with massive formiminoglutamic aciduria. Pediatric Research **9**: 117–122.

437 Frater-Schröder M, Hitzig WH, Grob DJ, Kenny AB, 1978. Increased unsaturated transcobalamin II in active autoimmune disease. *Lancet* **ii**: 238–239.

Index

199